Quality in General Practice

Katherine Birch
Research Fellow
Centre for Health Planning and Management
Keele University

Steve Field
Director of Postgraduate GP Education
NHSE, West Midlands

Ellie Scrivens
Professor of Health Policy
Centre for Health Planning and Management
Keele University

Foreword by
John Denham
Minister of State for Health

Radcliffe Medical Press

© 2000 Katherine Birch, Steve Field and Ellie Scrivens

Radcliffe Medical Press Ltd
18 Marcham Road, Abingdon, Oxon OX14 1AA

British Library Cataloguing in Publication Data

A catalogue record for this book is available from the British Library.

ISBN 1 85775 364 X

Typeset by Joshua Associates Ltd, Oxford
Printed and bound by TJ International Ltd, Padstow, Cornwall

Contents

Foreword

I believe that quality should be at the heart of primary healthcare. All patients who use the National Health Service are entitled to the highest quality of care regardless of where they live. Since being elected, the Government has put a great deal of effort and resources into ending the unacceptable variations in healthcare provision and into improving the quality of healthcare provided overall. The initiatives laid down in the *First Class Service* document are beginning to make an impact and the culture of clinical governance is pervading primary care.

Revalidation is on the horizon but it is important that all professionals and organisations within the NHS continue to critically examine how they provide care and develop systematic and comprehensive approaches to quality assurance now.

This book is intended to complement and reinforce the Department of Health's drive to improve quality. It discusses the key issues of quality review and performance assessment. It draws on a comprehensive national survey of all health authorities in England and Wales and provides practical examples of the breadth of quality and performance management programmes currently in use in primary care. It will provide an invaluable source of knowledge and experience to help professionals and their organisations reflect on their practice and develop a framework to improve the quality of healthcare that they provide.

John Denham MP
Minister of State for Health
June 2000

Acknowledgements

This book is based on part of a three-year research programme funded by the GP Unit, NHS Executive West Midlands, concerned with the management of quality and performance within general practice. We would like to pay particular thanks to all those health authorities who willingly shared their views and experiences with us, despite undergoing widespread organisational upheaval at the time and facing a battery of competing research demands. We would also like to thank Bill Poole and many of our colleagues who provided valuable support, criticisms and suggestions throughout. The views expressed here are those of the authors alone and not those of the NHS Executive.

Introduction

I will prescribe regimen for the good of my patients according to my ability and my judgement and never do harm to anyone. (Hippocratic Oath)

In the constantly changing environment of healthcare and consumerism, one thing is constant – the prevailing desire to protect the patient from harm. All medical practice should, as the Hippocratic Oath states, be for the benefit of patients and, at a broader level, the fundamental *raison d'être* of the NHS is to improve the physical and mental health of the population. But how do we know if the NHS is doing a good job? How can the public be assured that those practising medicine do so to a high standard and how can those providing healthcare demonstrate that they are delivering a quality service?

Within the healthcare arena, achieving a balance between the many related components which together assure the provision of a quality service is not always easy. Indeed, owing to the demands of modern medicine and the context within which it is delivered, one can argue that it is extremely difficult for the NHS to provide a high-quality, comprehensive service – particularly at an individual practitioner level. Whilst there is a general perception that 'all [professionals] want to practice well and seek to base their decisions and care on the best possible knowledge' (Roberts 1999), there are many practical difficulties associated with this. 'It has been estimated [for example] . . . that a doctor . . .

would need to read 19 articles every single day in a year just to keep abreast with the publications' (op. cit.). However, this is only one of many pressures felt by those working within the NHS.

With the rapid technological advances that have been made within medicine there is now the prospect of delivering healthcare in new ways, transcending both institutional and geographical boundaries (Rigby 2000). The limits of medicine are continually being challenged and we have seen major advances in knowledge, expertise and in the ways in which the NHS provides care. At the same time, the general public have become much more aware of, and knowledgeable about, health issues. Information about health – whether related to lifestyle, illness or the provision of NHS services (at a national, local or individual practitioner level) – now forms a part of everyday life. Furthermore, with recent develop-ments in telecommunications technology, people's ability to obtain global information about health issues (via the Internet, for example) has become almost limitless. This presents considerable challenges to those who deliver healthcare, since patients may use data from such sources to question decisions about their own care, without necessarily considering either the reliability of the informa-tion or its transferability to a UK context (Rigby 2000). Moreover, not only are practitioners having to respond to the opportunities and challenges brought about by new technologies, advancing knowledge and greater consumerism, but following media coverage of events such as the Bristol heart surgery cases in 1999, of the trial of Manchester GP, Dr Harold Shipman, in 2000 and of the pressures faced by an increasingly stretched NHS, there have been widespread calls for greater regulation of professional practice and improved performance of NHS services.

Reflective of the growing concerns about the provision of NHS services (Department of Health 1998a,b) and in order to demon-strate that the NHS is continuously striving to provide high-quality, accessible and effective healthcare, a range of new policies and procedures has been introduced. The Department of Health's consultation paper *Supporting Doctors, Protecting Patients* (DoH 1999c) has put the quality of patient care and the procedures for detecting and dealing with poor clinical performance at the very heart of the health agenda. Equally, all NHS organisations have been charged with continuously monitoring and developing the quality of the care that they provide. Recent service reorganisations have created new opportunities for all those involved in primary care to deliver care focused more specifically on the needs of local populations.

How then can those involved in primary care respond to such challenges? How can providers and commissioners demonstrate that the NHS is providing a high-quality service? How can the quality of organisational and individual performance be assessed and what are the main issues surrounding performance management in healthcare?

It is important that all those within the NHS critically examine how they provide care and develop a framework for assessing and monitoring both organisational and individual performance. Whilst clinical audit and critical event analysis have been increasingly used within general practice, there is a need to develop a more systematic and comprehensive approach to quality assurance – whether at a health authority, primary care trust, primary care group or individual practitioner level.

This book outlines the key issues connected with quality review and performance assessment, and is designed to be of benefit to all those concerned with the development of primary care. Based on the results of a national study of all health authorities (HAs) in England and Wales, it provides practical examples of the range of quality and performance management programmes currently in use within general practice and identifies the key questions which need to be addressed when developing such schemes. Whilst the principal focus is that of primary or practice-based care, many of the issues relating to quality and the assessment of individual and organisational performance are applicable across the whole of the NHS.

There are two main sections to the book:

Section I: A focus on quality reviews the emerging policy themes and considers the major issues involved when assessing quality or performance within any organisation. Specifically, different perspectives concerning 'quality' are outlined and contrasting systems of review and standards for assessment discussed.

Section II: Health authority performance review systems presents the results from the national survey of HAs and has three principal elements. Chapter 4 looks at the measures which have been introduced by HAs to support poorly performing general practitioners. Chapter 5 reviews the wide variety of schemes developed to assess the quality of general practice based care and draws together the major challenges facing those involved in performance management. Following the introduction of clinical governance, Chapter 6 outlines one approach which may be used to locate quality or performance management initiatives within a wider framework.

KB, SF and ES
June 2000

SECTION I

A focus on quality

Chapter 1

The NHS

More than 50 years after its inception, the NHS is experiencing a period of unparalleled pressure. This chapter outlines the factors which together have caused many to conclude that the NHS is in 'crisis' (BBC News, 6 January 1999), and briefly reviews some of the recent policy initiatives which have been introduced in an attempt to address these.

The 'new' NHS

Within modern societies, good health and a sense of well-being have generally come to be expected attributes of modern life. The rapid advancement of medical knowledge, technological developments and the position of the medical profession within our society have led to a common belief that most health problems can be treated through medical or surgical intervention (Morgan *et al.* 1985). Public knowledge about health matters has increased and expectations about what the NHS can and should provide have risen (DoH 1998a).

Set alongside such increased demands for service provision is the ever present problem of resourcing health services. A number of co-terminous 'external' socio-demographic and economic factors and 'internal' service-orientated developments have resulted in the NHS coming under increasing pressure (*see* Box 1.1). In the light of such factors, it became increasingly evident throughout the 1980s and 1990s that a substantial re-evaluation of healthcare policy and provision would be required (DoH 1989, 1997, 1998a,b). In response to calls for greater efficiency and improved effectiveness in the NHS, a range of service re-organisations has taken place

---

Box 1.1: Sources of pressure on the NHS

- Changes in population demography, whereby the average life expectancy has increased steadily throughout this century and now stands at 74.8 years for men and 80.1 years for women (1998). As a result 'elderly people (those aged 65 years and over) and, in particular, very elderly people (those aged 85 years and over) . . . continue to increase in number' (Annual Report, Chief Medical Officer, 1997).

- An increase in the prevalence of chronic diseases, disability and dependency which accompany such demographic changes.

- A reduction in the birth rate, which means that there are fewer people to look after the elderly and fewer workers to support them financially.

- Developments in clinical practice and advances in medical and information technology have led to changes in service provision (both in terms of the services provided and the mode of their delivery) and in both professional and public expectations about what the NHS can and should provide.

- Changing patterns of mortality and morbidity across all population groups.

- The persistence of inequalities in health between population groups (DHSS 1980, Acheson Report 1998) and criticisms concerning the effectiveness of NHS care.

- Increased awareness of health and healthcare issues which in turn has placed greater demands on those providing care to meet public expectations.

- Increased geographical mobility of the population and the decline of the extended family.

- Problems concerning the recruitment and retention of staff.

- A cash-limited service.

(e.g. DoH 1989, 1991, 1997, 1998a). However, it has been widely noted that 'as health care systems around the world undergo major reforms and [at the same time] resources remain limited, the quality of health care is threatened' (TPN 1998). Within the UK, for example, the development of the NHS 'internal market' and the ensuing emphasis that was placed by both purchasers and providers on aspects of contracting, such as costs and related activity, led to concerns about service quality being relegated to a poor third in terms of priorities (DoH 1998a,b, Paton *et al.* 1998).

Towards a primary care-led NHS

Throughout the 1990s there was a strategic shift in policy away from secondary care towards primary care and new ways of delivering and organising healthcare were sought. As a result, primary care – that is care predominantly provided by general practice, community nursing and psychiatric services, and the professions allied to medicine – has witnessed substantial changes to the ways in which services are organised, managed and delivered. These have included the relocation of some services away from the acute environment, the development of general practitioner fund-holding (GPFH) and the more recent introduction of primary care groups (PCGs) and primary care trusts (PCTs). Such changes have been brought about through a combination of factors. The value of supporting patients at home and providing care in a community setting has been identified as one way of alleviating the pressures on and costs of acute care, whilst from a commissioning perspective it has been argued that healthcare planning can best be achieved by those providers who are closest to patients. As a result, primary care providers have been given a much greater role in the planning and delivery of local healthcare.

Within the 'new' NHS, for example, PCGs have been established, bringing together groups of GP practices, and have been given a broad remit covering three salient areas.

- To improve the health of local population groups.
- To commission a range of services.
- To develop primary and community services.

However, as the DoH itself has previously acknowledged, giving primary care such a pivotal role is not without its problems.

> On the one hand, advances in medical knowledge backed up by new technologies and larger teams of dedicated staff have brought new skills to primary care and increasing investment has raised both the quality and the range of services provided. Additionally, through GP fundholding and GP-led commissioning many primary healthcare teams have taken on a wider role in the provision, planning and management of services. However, such changes and opportunities have also brought pressures on the service.
>
> Whilst services have generally improved, the effect has been patchy and what we now see is a situation whereby some parts of the country and some groups of people continue to be less well served by the NHS than others.

Equally, inequalities in health remain, and this holds true between different population groups (according to social class, gender and race) and between different locations (inner city and rural, north and south). Despite a range of policies which have sought to address the prevalence of health inequalities, these trends show no sign of abating (Acheson 1998).

Such disparity in the health status of the population and in the nature of service provision is problematic to a government committed to promoting good health and to ensuring equity of standards and access to healthcare services.

Focusing on quality

The Labour government has sought to place quality firmly at the heart of healthcare policy and practice. Moving away from a competitive, 'market-driven' model, with its overriding concern with costs and activity, a spirit of greater collaboration, openness and fairness has been encouraged.

> **Underlying and informing all relationships must be a fundamental shift in culture and behaviour away from the adversarial approach of the internal market.**

(NACGP 1997)

The Department of Health has reaffirmed the need for uniformity of standards throughout the *whole* of primary care, stating that 'services should not vary widely in range or quality in different parts of the country' (DoH 1997). The new emphasis:

> *shifts the focus onto quality of care so that excellence is guaranteed to all patients, and quality becomes the driving force for decision making at every level of the service . . . the new approach aims to improve standards of performance across the NHS.* (DoH 1998a)

It is envisaged that the way to achieving improved standards of service delivery is that of:

> *comparing performance and sharing best practice – not by financial competition between different parts of the service . . . the pursuit of quality and efficiency must go together if the NHS is to deliver the best for patients.* (DoH 1998a)

Such a reorientation of policy reflects a number of factors. Not only is the NHS having to respond to ever-increasing demographic and resource pressures, but within a wider context greater accountability and performance management have been called for throughout the whole of the public sector. PCGs, for example, are expected to have:

> *a rolling annual programme of action covering its three main functions (improving health and cutting*

health inequalities, commissioning services and developing
primary and community services), so that by 2002 all PCGs
*and primary care trusts are delivering **measurable***
improvements against their locally agreed milestones and
targets. (DoH 1998a)

For those working within primary or practice-based care, this
extended role and the emphasis which has been placed on
monitoring the quality of NHS care, brings with it the prospect
of significant changes to their pattern and orientation of work. For
example:

- there will be greater accountability and increased assessment of
  performance

- performance will be assessed, in part, in terms of quantifiable
  health gain across population/disease groups

- professionals will be required to demonstrate that they have
  undertaken programmes which ensure continuing professional
  development

- there will be a greater emphasis placed on evidence-based
  practice

- assessment of local health needs will play a major role in shaping
  local services, which in turn may lead to a development in the
  range and type of services provided within the practice

- there will be a greater focus on patient evaluation

- good communication across the whole of the practice team will
  be of paramount importance

- changing service configurations and the introduction of new
  technology into the healthcare environment may lead to shifting
  patterns of work.

In promoting and developing the quality of care provided,
particularly within a controlled budget, certain measures of monitoring quality are required. Historically, both those responsible for

purchasing or commissioning services and those responsible for providing healthcare have sought to define what is meant by 'quality' and have introduced ways to monitor and assess the standards of care provided and have developed strategies to improve service quality. Whilst the desire to promote the quality or performance of services is commendable, the emergence of a plethora of locally derived schemes with varying definitions of 'quality', foci, methodologies and outcome measures is problematic to a government committed to ensuring uniformity of standards throughout the NHS.

> *Considerable resources are being directed at the process of monitoring, and as each authority undertakes this activity independently, each is finding different solutions. Not only does this consume . . . resources, it also defects the quest for equity in quality which might be expected within a national health service.* (Scrivens 1995)

In striving to develop a more standardised approach to monitoring and developing the quality of care, a range of measures has been introduced. At a national level, legislation has been passed concerning standards of GP performance (the Medical Performance Act 1997) and several polices have been introduced which specifically relate to the performance management and quality assessment processes within the whole of the NHS. At a local level, HAs (together with representatives from other relevant bodies) are having to develop policies and procedures which address poor GP performance and PCGs also have a responsibility to review and develop the quality of primary care.

New legislation and new methods of assessing performance

Under the 1997 Medical (Professional Performance) Act, HAs are now able to refer cases of sub-standard medical performance to the

GMC if they believe such action to be necessary. Responsibility for monitoring GP performance falls to HAs, since they have a duty to 'provide support to GPs in . . . their primary care provision . . . through the provision of advice, investment and training' (EL (94) 79). This was underlined in the 1996 White Paper which emphasised the need for HAs to have 'clear arrangements to help identify inadequate performance by GPs' and encouraged 'the development of local arrangements for supporting doctors whose performance gives cause for concern through the issue of guidance . . . based on existing good practice and consultation with the profession'. The new legislation provides statutory powers to ensure that:

- doctors whose performance is alleged to be seriously deficient are assessed professionally

- when appropriate, doctors take remedial action if they wish to remain in practice

- where required, for the protection of the public, conditions regarding doctors' registration and practice can be imposed, including suspension from the GMC register.

The new performance procedures complement the existing 'fitness to practice' committees of the GMC and are designed to 'improve the quality of patient care by ensuring minimal standards of medical practice' (DoH Press Release, 20 May 1997). The aim of the new procedures is not 'to punish the doctor . . . but to assess whether performance [is] seriously deficient, through peer assessment and, if so, to try to improve that performance through counselling and retraining' (op. cit.).

Despite the prominent role which HAs have in addressing standards of professional performance, the nature of their relationship with GPs has been described as a 'complicating factor' in developing mechanisms to support GPs and in tackling issues of performance in general practice (ScHARR 1997). GPs are 'independent contractors, running what effectively amount to small businesses with the NHS as their main customer. There is therefore no conventional line of management [between GPs and HAs], and the nature of the relationship between a HA and the GPs in contract with it is necessarily subtle' (ScHARR 1997). Indeed, historically:

> GPs have enjoyed many of the freedoms of small businesses and incurred few of the risks. The virtual monopoly conferred by the registered list and referral system, together with a contract which until 1990 was simply tautologous, fostered in some GPs the worst excesses of small business untempered by the discipline of either market or public sector. (Huntington 1994)

Although the NHS (Primary Care) Act of 1997 offered the potential for the employment status of GPs to change, since it allowed for them to be directly employed by practices and trusts, the more conventional relationship between HAs and GPs remains the most common.

Within a wider quality management context, a number of policies have been introduced. The latest White Paper and consultation papers on a national framework for assessing performance outline a range of initiatives for developing quality within the NHS and for improving performance. National service frameworks have been developed for specific areas (e.g. coronary heart disease, mental illness) and new methods to assess how well the NHS is performing have been introduced, including national performance indicators (DoH 1997, 1998a,b, 1999a,b). These indicators are specifically designed to provide comparative information about the performance of hospitals and primary care providers in a number of key areas, and it is envisaged that these indicators will form a significant component of future quality review programmes.

However, one of the most far-reaching aspects of the government's new policy agenda is undoubtedly the introduction of clinical governance into the NHS (DoH 1997).

> Clinical governance is a framework through which all NHS
> organisations are accountable for continuously improving
> the quality of their services and safeguarding high standards
> of care by creating an environment in which excellence in
> clinical care will flourish.

Clinical governance places a statutory duty for quality improvement on all NHS organisations. It is based upon the ideas of corporate governance developed for the management and operation of company boards, successfully adopted by the NHS for the conduct of its trust and HA boards. The principles of clinical governance outlined by the government mean that all commissioners and providers will be required to monitor and develop the quality of care provided. Significantly, key individuals within NHS organisations have been made accountable for guaranteeing that clinical governance procedures are in place.

In order to ensure that appropriate quality improvement mechanisms exist throughout the NHS, an independent statutory body, the Commission for Health Improvement (CHI), has been established. The CHI has, as part of its remit, the power to independently assess local arrangements for the monitoring and development of quality. Alongside this, a special 'umbrella' HA has been created, the National Institute for Clinical Effectiveness (NICE), which will co-ordinate the functions of the National Prescribing Centre, the National Centre for Clinical Audit, the NHS Executive national guidelines and professional audit programmes. It will also cover effectiveness bulletins, a prescribers' journal and PRODIGY clinical guidance. The rationale for centralising these existing organisations is that NICE will provide a single focus for work promoting clinical cost effectiveness. NICE will also appraise and produce guidance on new and existing health interventions as well as producing audit methodologies. Information produced will be disseminated in two principal ways – through education and training of professionals, and through the production of appropriate patient information. Also contained within the overall national quality review programme is the development of a national survey of patient and user experience.

As a result of such initiatives, the status of 'quality' within the planning and delivery of healthcare has increased. However, transforming the rhetoric of clinical governance into reality represents a considerable undertaking. As Scally and Donaldson (1998) report, 'clinical governance is a big idea that has shown that it can inspire and enthuse. The challenge for the NHS – health professionals and managers alike – is to turn this new concept into reality.'

Overall therefore, the medical profession have increased powers of self-regulation and HAs have a greater role in assessing and monitoring both the performance of GPs and of local primary care services. At the same time, the NHS as a whole is seeking to standardise good practice through the establishment of the NICE and the CHI and to address issues of performance and quality improvement through clinical governance and national service frameworks.

In order to progress the new quality and performance management agenda, new relationships and methods of working will be required.

> *General practice must now recognise its changed relationships – both internally and externally. Primary care is fundamental to the relational challenge now facing the NHS. General practice in the early 1990s [was] particularly associated with a more politicised health care system into which the competitive contracting and marketing functions of a market were introduced. It justified its pivotal role in this by demonstrating a leading edge in terms of cost reductions, efficiency gains etc. Its future accountability within a more collaborative and controlled policy is likely to require a very different currency.* (Meads 1997)

The NHS guidance on clinical governance (DoH 1999a) provides both a vision and a framework for its implementation. In particular, it focuses on the need for improved *teamwork, partnership* and *communication* and outlines the responsibility of the primary care group to undertake four key implementation steps.

1   Establishing leadership, accountability and working arrangements.
2   Carrying out a baseline assessment of capacity and capability.
3   Formulating and agreeing a development plan in the light of such assessment.
4   Clarifying reporting arrangements within the board, with the production of annual reports.

The guidance allows for a high degree of freedom on how individual PCGs and, as some develop and attain trust status, PCTs implement the concept. It is therefore necessary for all those involved to consider how they approach assessments of quality and performance.

The consultation paper, *Supporting Doctors, Protecting Patients* (DoH 1999c), demonstrated the government's committment to ensuring that patients receive the best possible care available within the NHS. The context in which the paper was produced was one of increasing public concern triggered by high profile cases of poor clinical performance in the NHS. The trial of the Manchester GP, Dr Harold Shipman, for example, raised the profile of general practice and the position of single-handed GPs with their limited arrangements for formal peer review. The paper built upon the Department of Health's previous publications on quality and clinical governance and developed the proposed role of the new Commission for Health Improvement. The consultation paper generated a heated response from the general practice establishment because it challenged the concept of professional self-regulation, and raised serious questions about the NHS's own procedures for addressing poor clinical practice and their relationship to the

General Medical Council, the medical Royal Colleges and other professional bodies. It proposed to strengthen and co-ordinate the mechanisms to identify and prevent poor clinical performance and, in order to resolve cases of poor medical performance, suggested the establishment of a number of assessment centres. The document also proposed to make participation in medical audit compulsory for all GPs, as well as introducing a formal system of performance appraisal for all doctors, and suggested that the existing disciplinary procedures are replaced and new procedures devised in consultation with the profession. The aim of this was to ensure that HAs, PCGs and trusts have the same systems and procedures available to them as hospital trusts. This does, of course, raise profound questions about the status of the independent contractor.

The paper proposed three steps to the process for handling doctors whose performance causes concern (DoH 1999c).

1   When a problem arises at a local level, an initial review should take place to ascertain which of four categories the problem falls into: doubts or concerns about clinical performance (these would lead to a referral to an assessment and support centre); misconduct of a personal nature (which should be dealt with under the local employer's internal disciplinary procedures); failure to fulfil contractual commitments, such as failure to turn up for surgeries, failure to work as a member of the team (these would be dealt with under the employer's disciplinary procedures or contractual mechanisms); serious clinical problems or mistakes which warrant immediate referred to the GMC without taking the step of referral to the assessment and support centre.

2   The establishment of a number of assessment and support centres to provide impartial support to the doctor and HA, by advising on the action to be taken and to provide the doctor concerned with a supportive environment whilst undergoing assessment. The assessment may then result in a number of

outcomes which could include a period of re-education and training, re-skilling in a different field of medical practice, returning to practice under supervision, referral to the GMC, or referral for medical treatment.

3   The HA should take responsibility for implementing the findings of the assessment and support centre in each case.

It was envisaged that referral to one of these assessment and support centres would be rapid, with any retraining or skilling co-ordinated by the centre in close liaison with the HA.

The Department of Health claimed that these proposals would also allow a doctor, who wanted advice about an area of their practice, to self-refer. It is possible that the process would shorten the time spent in the existing procedures and reduce the need for legal involvement. It should also cut down on the inconsistencies of how problems are dealt with between different HAs and health boards throughout the UK, as demonstrated in this book.

Chapter 2

What is quality?

As the previous chapter outlined, quality has been placed at the very heart of Labour's health policy. But what is quality, how can it be measured and how can commissioners and providers build quality into their performance assessment programmes? Before reviewing the various methods that can be used to assess the quality of service provision, it is worth reflecting on the contrasting definitions, theories and concepts that can apply to the quality of practice-based care. This chapter explores professional, user (or public), managerial and political views concerning quality and considers which components of healthcare might form part of any quality or performance assessment process. It also reviews some of the wider issues surrounding 'quality', such as the requirement to have objectives for healthcare services in place before any assessment of service quality can be undertaken and the need to think about what the benefits of providing a quality service will be.

Quality: an unattainable ideal?

> There are those who believe that quality cannot be assessed [but] . . . it is important to establish that it is theoretically possible to evaluate quality; otherwise all effort will be in vain. The definition of quality states that it is a property of and judgement on care . . . The confusion over the nature of quality arises from the difficulty of explaining the reasons for the presence or absence of quality. (Baker 1992)

In developing and assessing the quality of NHS services, one immediately encounters a problem. There is no universal definition of quality, rather it has been used in a variety of ways (*see* Box 2.1). Quality is a complex issue and the contrasting definitions tend to reflect the concerns of various interest groups. The major stakeholders within healthcare often emphasise different components of a service and may also favour particular methods for reviewing and assessing the quality of care provided (e.g. the use of randomised control trials, in-depth interviews with users, economic evaluations of comparative treatments). For those involved in developing performance reviews or quality improvement schemes it is important

---

Box 2.1: Quality may be thought of in a variety of ways, for example:

- reducing variation in clinical practice, eliminating errors or poor practice

- short waiting times for elective surgery

- the patients' experience of the consultation which forms the basis of healthcare provision

- providing effective healthcare to different population groups

- 'that component of the difference between efficacy and effectiveness that can be attributed to care providers, taking account of the environment in which they work' (Brook and Lohr 1985)

- 'the expected ability of . . . care to achieve the highest net benefit according to the valuations of professions, individuals and society' (Baker 1992)

- 'the degree to which agreed standards are achieved and to which those standards are related to the highest priority requirements or needs of the users of the service given existing resource levels and other constraints' (CEPPP 1991)

- 'quality . . . depends essentially on access and on effectiveness: can patients get health care and is it any good when they get it?' (Roland *et al.* 1998)

to think about how, or indeed if, these various views can be amalgamated. We can all give an opinion about the quality of NHS care, but how and why we arrive at such a judgement depends upon our own views, expectations and knowledge base. Any quality review or performance assessment programme should therefore seek to capture this diversity of opinion whilst also ensuring that the correct policies and procedures are in place for effective and efficient service delivery. This multidimensional view of performance management is, of course, what clinical governance is all about.

There are four broad perspectives on quality, which may be categorised as:

- professional/medical

- lay

- managerial

- political.

Quality of professional practice

> Professional/medical quality is seen as the optimal healthcare given current biomedical knowledge.

Rigorous and visible self-regulation, together with continuing professional development, clinical guidelines and tools such as audit and critical event analysis are seen by the medical profession as the most appropriate means by which to ensure the standard of professional practice. The rationale for this rests on:

three pillars which together constitute the basis of [the profession's] independence or autonomy: expertise, ethics and service. Expertise derives from a body of knowledge and skills whose utility is constantly invigorated by the results of research. Ethical behaviour flows from a unique combination of values and standards. Service embodies a vocational commitment to put patients first. Independence gives individual doctors clinical freedom and the profession collectively the authority to decide about standards of professional practice and education and the organisation of medical work. (Irvine 1997)

Assessments in this context have largely been concerned with ensuring professional competencies and reviewing performance in relation to current standards, guidelines and protocols. Accordingly, the major areas for assessments of professional performance have traditionally been the highly technical or clinical aspects of service delivery (i.e. diagnosis, treatment, outcome) or those concerned with the management of the clinical environment.

However, the new climate of accountability and performance management means that the conduct and performance of professionals are becoming the subjects of considerable attention. One only has to recall the concerns raised by the Bristol heart surgery case and the media coverage of poor practitioner performance (e.g. Mr Melvyn Megitt, the NHS's highest paid dentist, who was struck off in September 1999 on the basis that 'he displayed a lamentable lack of skill, [and] . . . attempted to treat a grossly excessive number of patients for whom he failed to make adequate clinical notes' (General Dental Council Ruling, September 1999)) to realise that aspects of professional performance receive widespread and detailed coverage in the public arena. Whilst these may be relatively isolated incidents, the seriousness of the cases and the adverse publicity surrounding them means that the public are becoming increasingly aware of the standard of medical performance as a whole.

Both the medical profession and the professions allied to medicine are having to review their current arrangements for ensuring quality of professional practice and to develop and implement new forms of performance management to meet the demands of the new quality agenda. In the absence of, until recently, any moves to implement professional recertification or revalidation, calls for the improved performance management of doctors have grown. A succession of commentaries by the President of the GMC highlighted that the profession itself was acutely aware of the need to ensure standards of medical performance:

> *there are still criticisms that we [the medical profession] seem reluctant to assure doctors' competence and protect patients from poor practice. There are also criticisms that we are not addressing the widespread dissatisfaction with the attitude of some doctors, including their paternalism and poor communication with both patients and colleagues and are failing to make self-regulation demonstrably effective and responsive.* (Irvine 1997)

In response to criticisms about the nature of self-regulation, the GMC sought to promote a more visible system of review, and the new legislation concerning medical performance gave HAs and the GMC additional powers to review the performance of those doctors deemed to be failing.

More recently, and in what represents a complete volte-face regarding assessments of medical competencies, the GMC have endorsed key recommendations for the implementation of revalidation for all registered doctors. The move represents 'the biggest shake up in the regulation of the profession since the NHS was founded in 1948' (Irvine 1999b), although a model for revalidation will not come into effect before 2001 and it will be several years after this before a national system of revalidation is up and running. Under the new plans there will be a link between a doctor's performance in any assessment and their registration to practise. The measures will cover GPs and hospital specialists to begin with, but will eventually include all doctors. All doctors will have to submit to local and national assessments and such reviews will 'include evidence of keeping up to date and other matters. The contents would be for more detailed examinations, but there would be a profile of that doctor and that profile would trigger revalidation on the register' (Irvine 1999b). What is not clear at the moment is what aspects of performance will be subject to assessment, what the process of assessment will be and how such a task will be organised and resourced.

Establishing a coherent and acceptable programme of revalidation may prove difficult, as previous attempts to determine quality of professional practice have highlighted significant differences within and between the professions.

> *One of the characteristic weaknesses of improving quality within the NHS has been the insistence of each main profession or specialty on developing its own systems rather than co-operating to produce a co-ordinated and comprehensive strategy.* (CEPPP 1991)

The new performance procedures and the requirements of clinical governance mean that performance review strategies will have to be introduced and developed well before the moves to implement professional revalidation are completed – although it is to be hoped that the latter will look at the considerable work already undertaken to identify and support poor GP performance. In the immediate future, the challenge is to develop systems which demonstrate that the correct polices and procedures are in place in order to safeguard standards of professional practice and to ensure that poor performance is detected.

One of the problems in developing any review of professional performance is deciding which aspects of performance are subject to review and who decides what the appropriate standards or definitions of quality of care are. Traditionally, 'good' professional performance has been determined from within the profession, since it has previously been argued that only those with specialist training and knowledge are in a position to assess medical performance. More recently, as illustrated by central policy, there has been a call to incorporate other views on quality into the equation, most notably those of the patient.

Quality from a lay/patient perspective

> Lay or user views about quality relate to the way in which care is provided as well as the outcomes of such care.

Missing from all but a handful of studies [of quality] is the essential first step . . . recognition of the patients' problems and needs. Almost all studies of quality of care start with a diagnosis, a suspected diagnosis or a particular indicated preventative intervention and evaluation of care is directed at that particular condition. This is a professionally specified definition of patients' needs, not a patient specific definition . . . Study designs that start with patient-defined problems and follow them through diagnosis, management, treatment and outcomes assessment are an important complement to . . . strategies that are professionally focused. (Starfield 1998)

Quality of care from a lay or patient perspective is derived from a personal assessment of the care that is provided (which may include both technical and interpersonal aspects) and may or may not be associated with health outcomes. Quality from this viewpoint might therefore relate to a number of different features of healthcare delivery. These may include access to healthcare services, information provision and communication, waiting times, pain relief and improved health status. The degree to which people rate the care that they receive also depends upon their previously held assumptions about healthcare and the extent to which they feel that such care meets their own self-perceived needs.

The methods used to assess the quality of NHS care from a patient perspective have tended to fall into one of two broad categories.

1   Studies which seek to assess how satisfied patients were with the care (or components of care) received.
2   More in-depth studies (using both qualitative and quantitative methods) which focus on areas such as the illness experience, perceived need and attitudes towards the services provided.

Both of these have their value, although it is important for those committed to improving the quality of service provision from the patient's perspective to consider not only how satisfied patients are with the care that they receive, but also to examine how *important* different aspects of care are to a particular patient group. Patients may be very satisfied with an aspect of care which they do not regard as being very important and, equally, may be very dissatisfied with the care provided in an area of high importance to them. The 'gap' between satisfaction and salience may have a profound effect on patient's evaluation of service provision, especially if services are not providing what patients feel that they need (Poole and Birch 1997).

From a quality perspective, user evaluations may present problems in developing services, since what individuals feel that they want from services may not necessarily be what they are judged to medically need nor may it be possible to meet their demands within local constraints. Equally, different groups of patients or individual patients within various patient or population groups may define quality differently or have contrasting perceptions of service provision. However, providing services which take into account user views is important; high levels of patient satisfaction can have a number of benefits. These include, *inter alia*, greater adherence to treatment regimes (Daltroy and Liang 1991) and lower levels of anxiety (Poole and Birch 1997) which in turn can have a positive effect on the health status of the individual (Teixeira *et al.* 1999).

The new PCGs will both provide and commission a range of services for and on behalf of their patients. As with GPFH, this places them in a potentially unique position to offer primary and secure acute care which meets the needs of distinct population groups. There is, therefore, a responsibility on commissioners at a PCG level (as well as HAs) to not only review their own services, but also to assess the response of patients to the care that they commission. However, with user involvement having achieved what can only be described as a limited or patchy impact on the delivery of NHS services in the past, the challenge now is to develop mechanisms which incorporate the views of those who receive care into overall quality assessment and quality improvement programmes.

Managerial and political views on quality

Definitions of managerial quality have traditionally tended to focus on the use of resources (both human and non-human) and the activity which is achieved for such inputs. From a wider, political viewpoint, quality has related to activity and cost issues, with sporadic initiatives such as the Patient's Charter and drives to reduce waiting times. More recently the DoH has outlined a particular view of quality with which all NHS organisations will have to comply.

> *Every part of the NHS and everyone who works in it should take responsibility for working to improve quality. This must be quality in its broadest sense: doing the right thing, at the right time for the right people and doing them right – first time. And it must be the quality of the patient's experience as well as the clinical result – quality measured in terms of prompt access, good relationships and efficient administration.* (DoH 1997, para 2.12)

This 'right first time' view of quality will be determined by:

* timely access to care
* high-quality clinical care

- high-quality interpersonal care

- efficient administration and management.

In assessing quality, it is important to note that the new political definition of quality places the patient's experiences on an equal footing with clinical quality. It has only been with the increased consumerism of modern-day life and the calls for greater account-ability in the public sector that the voice of the patient has been accorded more significance. Previously, the medical or professional perspective concerning the provision of NHS care has tended to dominate, irrespective of whether the users of such a service were critical of the care that was provided. Indeed, in some areas, such as maternity care, there was a profusion of evidence – built up over a considerable period of time – to suggest that existing patterns of NHS care required reform. In the face of resistance from the medical profession however, it was not until the early 1990s, when a House of Commons Health Committee Review recommended widescale shifts in the philosophy and practice of maternity care, that such changes were made (Birch 1997; House of Commons Health Committee Report, Maternity Services 1992).

The publication of the Department of Health consultation paper, *Supporting Doctors, Protecting Patients* (DoH 1999c), put the quality of care provided by GPs right at the centre of the national debate on standards of NHS care. Its publication came at a sensitive time for the NHS with the on-going enquiry into the Bristol tragedy and the trial of the Manchester GP, Dr Harold Shipman. The enormous publicity that was generated by such cases focused attention on the effect of poor medical care on patients and their families. The Secretary of State in his foreword suggested that there should be systems in place to help the small minority of doctors whose performance gives cause for concern, and that the inflex-ibility of the existing arrangements should be reviewed. The consultation document raised several important questions about the effectiveness of professional self-regulation and the ability of the diverse medical bodies who undertake aspects of regulation to effectively protect patients from the minority of underperforming doctors. The paper alludes to the General Medical Council's development of systems for revalidation but the issues raised in the paper draw into focus the question of whether the General Medical Council can continue with its central and independent role in the self-regulation of the profession.

The Commission for Health Improvement appears to be gearing itself up for an important role in monitoring organisational quality, identifying poor performance, and ensuring that systems of clinical governance are in place and working effectively within each of the individual practices that make up PCGs and trusts. It is clear, therefore, that the monitoring of quality and arrangements for dealing with poor clinical performance will be the subject of a great deal of government attention to ensure that the health service provides the very highest quality of patient care possible.

Synthesising views

Within the new climate of performance management and clinical governance, it is essential to ensure that quality programmes bring together the range of views outlined.

- Quality from a *patient* perspective typically relates to access, responsiveness, good inter-personal communication, information provision, appropriate treatment, relief of symptoms and improvement in health status.

- Quality from a *professional* point of view includes ensuring the technical competencies of staff, reviewing medical practice (through, for example, training, continuing professional development and medical audit), autonomous practice, achieving desired outcomes and continually seeking to expand the limits of medical knowledge through the appropriate means.

- Quality from a *management/commissioning* perspective incorporates factors such as the most appropriate use of resources, ensuring that the care provided is of a high quality, risk management, and developing services to take into account changes in both the 'external' and 'internal' environment.

(adapted from Irvine and Irvine 1996)

The diversity of opinion as to what constitutes quality in the NHS reflects both the wide range of different groups involved in the provision of NHS care and also the various components which might form the basis for performance assessment programmes. The actual location and range of services, the manner in which they are provided, the skills and expertise of those providing care, the technical facilities available, waiting times, cost per case, outcomes and whether the professionals involved are committed to a programme of lifelong learning are all possible aspects of any review programme. It is necessary therefore not only to achieve a balance between the various perspectives concerning service provision but to develop these within a framework which systematically looks at the ways in which services are provided.

The components of quality care

Within any performance review or quality improvement programme there needs to be a focus for assessment. In determining the various components of care, services have traditionally been broken down into two broad sections – those areas which are concerned with the technical or organisational side of service delivery and those which focus on the interpersonal nature of professional/patient encounters or on inter-professional relationships. These have commonly been subdivided into aspects of structure, process and outcome (Donabedian 1980).

Structure

In assessments of service provision, structure is generally used to refer to the available facilities and equipment together with the organisational infrastructure supporting care provision (i.e. what is in place). Aspects of service provision which fall under the remit of structure would include, for example, the quality of the practice premises, the type of equipment used, the staffing structure (e.g. medical, professions allied to medicine) and medical records systems. Whilst there may not necessarily be a relationship between structure, care provision and outcome, it is obviously more difficult for high-quality care to be delivered if there are major failings in the structural aspects of the organisation.

Process

This refers to how care is provided and may include a whole raft of performance dimensions such as number and length of consultations, tests conducted, communication between health professionals in the practice, links to other providers, the doctor/patient encounter and prescribing habits. Aspects of performance may be modified in the light of personal knowledge, experience or product availability (as in the use of generic drugs or new technologies which offer alternative methods of working) or may be influenced by external factors (such as the informed patient). Many quality schemes focus on the process aspects of service provision since they are often quantifiable or recorded (e.g. patterns of prescribing) and may be compared to norms for particular aspects of care provision (e.g. generic prescribing rates).

Outcome

Reviewing the performance of NHS providers through a comparative assessment of key outcome indicators is a central feature of the new performance strategies. Data on a whole range of outcomes (e.g. hospital mortality rates, readmissions) are now collected and published, the rationale for this being that if this type of information is publicly available it will allow providers to compare their performance with others. Such data are also freely accessible to the general public. One only has to look at the BBC website, for example, to see a number of pages devoted to recent NHS performance indicators.

Controversy and debate over the use of outcome indicators to assess individual and collective performance abound, the reasons being that 'outcomes of care are conceptualised in different ways . . . death, disease, disability, discomfort and dissatisfaction . . . [and] developing valid measures of outcome is one of the major research challenges in general practice today' (Irvine and Irvine 1996). The problem of looking solely at outcome measures is compounded by the whole question of *attribution* – how do the various factors or inputs of care combine to produce a particular outcome? Health outcomes may be influenced by a range of factors, such as underlying health, clinical skill, patterns of care and socio-demographic and environmental factors, and it is often difficult to associate an outcome with a specified clinical (or related) input. One can, of course, conclude that a particular package of care resulted in a net benefit of 'x', but there are a number of individuals and services which combine to produce this. Equally, the outcomes of any package of care may be dependent upon patients following the prescribed treatment programmes and taking medication correctly. Whilst good communication between the practitioner and the client may influence treatment and prescription adherence, health outcomes themselves may be outside the control of those providing care (Giuffrida *et al.* 1999).

It is also the case that outcome indicators may not adequately capture the pattern of care received by particular patient groups. This is illustrated by the case of Weston Park Hospital in Sheffield, a specialist cancer centre which treats many patients in the terminal stages of their illness. Following publication of the first perform-ance indicator tables on mortality, the hospital had a high number of patients who died shortly after emergency surgery. However, further investigation revealed that the hospital does not carry out a single operation (cited on the BBC health web pages, referenced September 1999).

Notwithstanding such problems, outcomes have been given a central role in the new performance assessment framework. No longer will it be acceptable just to look at *how* things are done within the NHS, although this may be easier than looking at outcomes. The achievements and impact of care will have to be taken into account in any evaluations of NHS services.

The concept of assessing care in terms of structure, process and outcome was advanced by Maxwell (1984). He considered what the various components of quality might be, and this was later extended to include questions that might enable service providers and users to assess the services provided (*see* Table 2.1).

Objectives for care

When looking to develop a quality review programme, it is essential to ask the question 'what is the service, intervention, or treatment supposed to achieve?', since without defined objectives it is impossible to decide if care has been successful.

Service quality should not be a matter of vague aspirations and warm rhetoric. Before the concept can be made operational it is necessary to have clear requirements and then develop standards for meeting each of them.

(CEPPP 1991)

Developing objectives for healthcare is particularly problematic, not least because of the various interest groups involved. Essentially, however, there are two interrelated steps to defining the objectives for a service. Initially, agreement has to be reached about what the various components of care are and what 'good' or 'high' quality is relative to these. Secondly, it is vital to have clearly stated goals or objectives relating to the services provided. These might

Table 2.1   Looking at service quality (Maxwell 1984)

Aspects of quality	Questions that enable an assessment of quality to be made
Effectiveness	Is the treatment given the best available in a technical sense, according to those best equipped to judge? What is their evidence? What is the overall result of the treatment?
Acceptability	How humanely and considerately is this treatment/service delivered? What does the patient think of it? What would/does an observant third party think of it? What is the setting like? Are privacy and confidentiality safeguarded?
Efficiency	Is the output maximised for a given input or (conversely) is the input minimised for a given level of output? How does the unit cost compare with the unit cost elsewhere for the same treatment/service?
Access	Can people get this treatment/service when they need it? Are there identifiable barriers to services (e.g. distance, inability to pay, waiting lists, waiting times) or is there a straightforward breakdown in supply (rationing of some treatments according to location)?
Equity	Is this patient or group of patients being fairly treated relative to others? Are there any identifiable failings in equity (on the grounds of socio-economic group, race, treatment group for example)?
Relevance	Is the overall pattern and balance of services the best that could be achieved, taking into account the needs and wants of the population as a whole?

take the form of organisationally specific objectives (e.g. access, equity) or might relate to the treatment of specific patient groups. Equally, quality reviews should not only assess service provision against stated objectives, but should also ask whether such objectives are appropriate for that particular organisation or locality.

Collective responsibility

In assessing the quality of any care programme, one immediately encounters a major problem – that of whether assessments should focus on the performance of individual practitioners, collective practice (i.e. the practice, primary care team or professional group), the organisations within which they work or all of these. Healthcare services are integrated systems of care processes, rather than organised as independent and unrelated services. The relationships between individual providers of care, the structures and organisations within which they work, the socio-demographic characteristics of the local population and the quality and outcomes of patient care are all interrelated, and are therefore central to the quality debate.

Key issue

What is the relationship between the performance of an individual, the performance of a team, the organisational infrastructure within which care is delivered, the demographic characteristics of the local poulation and health outcomes?

The need for a multifarious view of quality can be seen through an examination of how attitudes towards quality management have changed. Typically, management of healthcare quality was based on the assumption that the outcome of patient care in terms of health status was down to the actions of individual clinicians. However, during the 1980s the view emerged that the outcome of patient care was in fact a result of the clinician interacting with the healthcare environment and management systems, both organisational and clinical, which were in place. Managers could no longer assume that poor clinical results were always down to poor clinical practice. Clinicians operate within complex systems which affect their actions. Most management models therefore begin by assessing the organisational systems and processes used. They are based on the understandable assumption that quality of professional practice would be improved if the organisation was well-ordered, ensuring access to medical records, appropriate diagnostic testing and support, and good staffing (Roberts *et al.* 1984). This multidimensional approach (focusing on both clinical skills and the organisational context within which care is delivered) has emphasised the need to understand the complex systems involved in the delivery of healthcare. More importantly, it has suggested that failure in terms of patient care is due not only to individual clinician failure, but also the failure of the system within which they work. Frequently cited in this context is the Pareto assumption of quality – 80% of things that go wrong are due to a system rather than to an individual. But the system in question is not simply that of organisation – it may be inappropriate training or a lack of training; it may be a lack of human resource management to appoint appropriately qualified staff; it may be the lack of proper audit systems to check on activities (Scrivens 1995). The importance of this 'systems' approach to thinking about quality cannot be over emphasised. As Øvretveit (1999) highlights, in a study of hospital care in Norway,

> *every day . . . on average 3 people are likely to die unnecessarily because of poor quality hospital care. 45% of patients experience some 'medical mismanagement' and 17% suffer events which lead to a longer stay or more serious problems . . . Only 8% of anaesthetic errors were found in a recent study to be due to human error – 92% were due to 'system' errors.*

Clinical governance places a responsibility on all organisations, whether commissioner or provider, to review quality. Covering all aspects of care and all areas of NHS services, it encompasses those individual, collective and organisational factors which contribute

---

Box 2.2: Healthcare as a system

Quality assessments might consider individual, collective and organisational aspects such as:

- infrastructure (management, systems, policies and procedures, team structures and relationships, staffing ratios)

- superstructure (buildings, capital replacement, upgrading, equipment)

- education (professional assessment, mentoring, continuing professional development

- quality assurance (audit procedures, review mechanisms)

- practice population characteristics (age, deprivation, ethnicity, etc.).

---

to healthcare provision in an effort to ensure that the right thing is done, at the right time and in the right way – and it is done right first time (*see* Box 2.2).

The RCGP perspective on quality

The UK currently has no system of professional re-certification or revalidation, whereby a doctor's competency to practice is examined on a regular basis (unlike other countries such as Canada and Australia)[1]. Instead, attention has tended to focus more on self-regulation, on developing continuing professional development (through education) programmes and on recognising cases of high-quality performance. The RCGP schemes which acknowledge high-quality professional care are a useful reference for those wishing to develop quality schemes, since they provide an outline

[1] As indicated earlier, new proposals have been outlined by the GMC, supported by other medical bodies, to strengthen procedures for professional self-regulation through a process of revalidation. A model for revalidation will be developed by 2001, although until then the current arrangements for professional self-regulation, clinical audit and local governance will act as the main safeguards of professional standards.

of what one of the major professional organisations regard as good quality general practice.

Individual GPs can seek to become Members of the RCGP and, later, Fellows of the RCGP[2]. Fellowship by Assessment is achieved following both a written submission and assessment of consulting skills (submitted on video) and a visit to the applicant by three assessors. The assessment process is based upon evidence relating to the following detailed set of criteria, which covers both clinical skills and organisational structures and processes.

- Basic qualification and membership of RCGP
- Availability

- Consultation skills (video and documentary evidence)
- Clinical care

- General input into practice development
- Continuity of care

- The consultation and the organisation of care
- Health promotion

- Out-of-hours emergency care
- Records/registers

- Premises and equipment
- Teamwork

- The social dimension
- Resources

- Communication with patients
- Future planning

Both Membership and Fellowship schemes are regarded as promoting 'Gold' standards within the profession (Moore 1996).

Whilst the Fellowship by Assessment does not directly examine the outcomes of care, a major part of the assessment process focuses on the clinical skills of the applicant – through both direct observation and retrospective analysis of care notes (under the category of 'clinical care'). The organisational structures and processes which impact on patient care also form an integral part of the assessment,

[2] Fellowship can either be attained through nomination or by assessment.

covering aspects such as prescribing, out-of-hours care and premises. The assessors may also consider the views of other practice staff.

Membership of the RCGP has traditionally been achieved by examination. However, reflective of the growing concern to assess performance in practice, Membership by Assessment of Performance (MAP) was introduced in the summer of 1999 following extensive consultation and piloting. It is intended to offer a new route to membership of the RCGP for experienced GPs who can show evidence of good-quality everyday practice. MAP is based on the principle that many established GPs prefer to demonstrate good practice through compilation of written, oral and video material to be assessed by their peers rather than by sitting a traditional examination. They will also have to submit a videotape of their own consultations to be assessed alongside those sitting the MRCGP examination. While the assessment is of the individual doctor, rather than the practice, it is anticipated that in many practices partners will work together towards the assessment and this should lead to an increase in reflective practice and in the quality of care provided by the practices themselves.

In addition to Membership and Fellowship of the RCGP, some practices seek to attain 'accredited status' as a training practice for GP registrars. This form of accreditation is professionally orientated and responsibility for its operation is devolved to Regional General Practice Education Committees. It should not be confused with those accreditation schemes which focus on the overall quality of care provided by an institution (or part thereof) or on the organisational aspects of care. The various schemes are distinct and operate for different purposes (although there may be some overlap regarding those aspects of service provision which form the basis of assessment).

Professional accreditation for training purposes

In 1976, the Joint Committee for Postgraduate Training for General Practice (JCPTGP) was founded from a working partnership that had grown between the two main bodies representing family doctors in the UK – The Royal College of General Practitioners (RCGP) and the General Medical Services Committee (GMSC) of the British Medical Association (BMA).[3] Today, membership of the JCPTGP also includes representatives from other organisations who have an interest in general practice training. The Committee is an independent body which works to provide high standards of training, education and support for GP registrars. The Committee's main responsibilities are:

- to set standards of general practice training throughout the UK and the armed services, including supervision of training and monitoring the performance of Deaneries[4] in providing training programmes

- to approve posts for use in general practice training

- to issue certificates of prescribed and equivalent experience to doctors who satisfactorily complete training in general practice

- to issue certificates of acquired rights

- to act as the competent authority in the UK for the purposes of Title IV of the Council Directive 93/16/EEC which deals with the arrangements for training and employment of GPs in the European economic area.

In practice the responsibility for trainer selection is devolved to the Deanery or Regional General Practice Education Committees. The criteria for training practice selection are defined regionally in line with the national JCPTGP guidelines. Furthermore, the JCPTGP visit each of the Deaneries every three years to ensure that the standards of training in the Deanery fulfil the national and regional

---

[3] The GMSC is now known as the General Practice Committee of the BMA.
[4] A Deanery is the geographical area for which a Dean of Postgraduate Medical and Dental Education is responsible. In England, there may be two or three Deaneries in any one NHSE region, with the exception of the West Midlands where there is one Deanery.

criteria. The following section outlines the criteria by which individuals and practices are assessed as potential trainers within the West Midlands.

1 The trainer as a doctor

The Trainer must:

1.1   normally be a principal in general practice
1.2   normally have three years' experience of general practice after completing vocational training
1.3   be physically and mentally fit to teach
1.4   be committed to providing comprehensive and continuing quality care and services to patients. This should include setting an example of enthusiasm, competence, good patient care, good practice organisation and the ability to use limited resources effectively
1.5   ensure that clinical work outside the practice and the time spent in contributing to local or national organisations does not interfere with their time for contact with patients or for teaching
1.6   be prepared and able to show the quality of his/her practice
1.7   be available to patients by an efficient system of surgery consultations, home visiting and out-of-hours care so that the Registrar has experience of all of these aspects
1.8   be aware that the Registrar should have experience of being on call through the night, assessing and responding to calls from patients. They must maintain cover for the Registrar either by the Trainer or another named doctor within the practice. Use of a deputising service or a co-operative is acceptable
1.9   be able to communicate with patients and all those working with them and should be willing to illustrate their consulting skills with videotaped consultations. They should be able to

demonstrate an ability to analyse a consultation and teach consultation skills to their Registrar

1.10 keep up to date with current medical care by attending sessions of continuing personal development and be familiar with current medical literature, particularly the literature of general practice

1.11 have academic credibility. New trainers must have attained the MRCGP

1.12 demonstrate a commitment to the professional guidance contained within the GMC publications *Good Medical Practice* and *Maintaining Good Medical Practice*

1.13 be able to demonstrate involvement with clinical governance.

2 The Trainer as a teacher

The Trainer must:

2.1 have enthusiasm for teaching

2.2 have satisfactorily completed a preparatory trainers' course and a foundation course recognised as appropriate by the West Midlands Deanery

2.3 attend the local trainers' workshop

2.4 attend, three days' training accredited by the Deanery GP Education Committee (DGPEC) and five days' training accredited by the AGPEC (Association of GPEC) averaged over five years

2.5 be willing to be assessed and able to demonstrate their development as a teacher

2.6 follow the Deanery protocol for the appointment of Registrars

2.7 organise teaching in the practice and produce a training programme appropriate to the Registrar's needs at the beginning of the year

2.8 assess the Registrar's knowledge, skills and attitudes on a regular basis and keep a written record of their progress using the appropriate assessment folder from the Deanery's resource pack; Trainers must keep a copy of the assessment package for future reference for each of their registrars

2.9 be able to demonstrate their ability to:
(a) identify the Registrar's learning needs
(b) implement strategies to address these needs
(c) appropriately address the achievement of these needs

2.10 work with the primary healthcare team to provide an appropriate teaching programme. This will involve at least three hours of undistributed teaching time a week. This time should include formal tutorials, case analysis, and discussions. They must use a variety of teaching techniques including topic teaching, random and problem case analysis, video recording and role play, clinical case presentations, projects and research work. The Trainer must produce a recent video of a tutorial for the purpose of reapproval

2.11 ensure that other practice partners and members of the practice team are involved in the teaching programme, the Trainer maintaining overall responsibility for the management of this programme

2.12 arrange visits to places of interest including other practices. This should address the needs of the new NHS, such as experience of inner city practice

2.13 ensure that the Registrar keeps an educational log

2.14 keep a separate educational log of activities involving the Registrar

2.15 ensure that the Registrar is actively involved in the primary healthcare team. Their workload should not exceed that of the average partner's workload.

2.16 maintain cover at all times for the Registrar either personally or by arranging cover with a named partner within the practice. A single-handed Trainer if absent from the practice must arrange cover with a neighbouring Trainer

2.17 encourage the Registrar to be responsible for their own continuing education and to facilitate the Registrar's progress through formative and summative assessment

2.18   ensure that the Registrar has practical experience of evidence-based practice including clinical audit in a general practice setting and must ensure that the Registrar produces an audit project during the practice year

2.19   encourage the Registrar to attend the half-day release course and any other courses relevant to their needs

2.20   obtain information concerning the Registrar's attendance at the half-day release course. (The Course Organiser will send an attendance record at the half-day release course at least twice a year to the Trainer). Regular or excessive absences must be discussed by the Trainer with the Registrar. The Area Director must be informed

2.21   contact the local Course Organiser and seek further guidance from the Area Director if the Registrar's progress proves to be unsatisfactory

2.22   use any appropriate information gained in the summative assessment process to inform their decision on signing a certificate of satisfactory completion (VTR/1); this is an essential criteria for the approval and re-approval of trainers

2.23   encourage the Registrar to take the membership examination of the Royal College of General Practitioners and to help the Registrar to prepare for it

2.24   periodically participate as a member of the AGPEC visiting team.

3 The training practice

Although trainers are appointed as individuals, the DGPEC supports the concept of the training practice where all members take part in the teaching process.

3.1   (a) single-handed practices are also appointed as training practices. Singled-handed trainers may only appoint a full-time registrar for a six-month period. A part-time registrar may be appointed

(b) in single-handed practices the registrar may not act as a locum for the Trainer when the Trainer is away on holiday or ill

(c) in single-handed practices, when the Trainer is absent, the Trainer must arrange an educational programme with advice from a named general practitioner with educational experience from a neighbouring practice

3.2   proposed significant changes within the practice affecting staffing, partners and premises should be notified in writing to the Area Director

3.3   there must be good relationships and good communication between all members of the practice team

3.4   there must be good organisation within the practice and this should include ready availability of doctors through a flexible appointment system. There should be justifiable policies for home visiting, out-of-hours calls and prescribing

3.5   the practice must be able to demonstrate activities consistent with a functional primary healthcare team

3.6   the practice must provide a contract and job description for all employees. This includes a registrar who should be provided with a contract

3.7   the practice should provide help for the Registrar regarding accommodation, telephone and other allowances payable under the NHS provision

3.8   a written practice guide must be provided for the Registrar

3.9   the practice should assist the Registrar in finding a suitable post at the end of the training year

3.10   the practice annual report should include a section on its educational activities

3.11   the list size of the practice should be of an appropriate size for teaching

3.12   the practice premises should be of an appropriate size for training. The Registrar should have priority use of their own room

3.13   the practice should possess a comprehensive range of equipment for modern general practice. The Registrar should be provided with a medical bag and all necessary equipment and drugs on joining the practice

3.14 the Training Practice must own and provide video equipment for teaching purposes

3.15 records must be available for all patient contacts including home visits. The records must have the following:

3.16 all medical records and hospital correspondence must be filed in practice notes in date order. The records must contain a relevant medical summary of important past illnesses and there should be a demonstrable structure for keeping such information up to date. Appropriate medical records must contain easily discernible drug therapy lists for patients on long-term therapy. These criteria apply whether the records are in manual or computerised form. The practice must have methods for monitoring prescribing habits as an important part of the audit process

3.17 disease register must be up to date and in use. The practice should be able to demonstrate recall systems for regular reviews of patients with chronic disorders or those who need regular screening

3.18 there must be full access to general practice journals, literature and other authoritative sources of knowledge available at the practice premises, with adequate instructions and cataloguing

3.19 the practice must demonstrate that the audit mechanism is being taught. There should be a core programme covering practice access, clinical effectiveness and risk management, all of which will be monitored at the practice visit

3.20 the consultation rate of the practice should allow optimal consulting which would normally for the Registrar be not more than one patient every ten minutes

3.21 the practice must be on the internet and have an e-mail address (by 2000).

(NHSE, West Midlands)

For any PCG or practice wishing to review the quality of care provided, the criteria outlined above are significant, since they broadly represent the professional view as to what constitutes good-quality practice in general practice.

The benefits of quality care

Whilst the benefits of promoting quality and maintaining high standards of professional practice may seem obvious (*see* Box 2.3), measuring the impact of any initiative and assessing the respective improvement in terms of service quality, performance and health improvement may not be an easy task.

Box 2.3: The benefits of quality care

- Applying up-to-date professional techniques and knowledge (through continuing professional development) is in the best interests of both the patient and the practitioner.

- Moving towards greater standardisation of access and professional practice leads to equity of provision.

- In a resource-limited service, achieving, improving and promoting efficiency is desirable (through, for example, generic prescribing, incorporating economic evaluations into assessments of healthcare provision).

- Improving the quality of care (through better communication, for example) may lead to higher levels of patient satisfaction and compliance.

- Sound quality review and audit mechanisms ensure that account-ability is visible and risk management practised.

- Improved staff morale may in turn may lead to greater teamwork-ing and innovation.

  The increasing emphasis on quality has very positive implications for the staff of these services. If you are a doctor, nurse . . . it is unlikely that you are going to be wholly satisfied with talk of economy and efficiency. One of the chief motivations of many such staff is to improve the quality

---

> *of the service they provide . . . so a programme for quality improvement*
> *can enhance staff morale as well as raising the satisfaction levels of those*
> *who use the service.* (CEPPP 1991)
>
> • Increased satisfaction amongst users may have a range of positive
>   benefits – increased adherence to treatment regimes, more appro-
>   priate utilisation of health services in the future, less anxiety.

Following the development of any performance assessment programme or the introduction of a quality improvement programme,
it is important that the impact of such a process – whether at an
individual practitioner level or in terms of the impact on services or
population – is assessed. This requires both an appreciation of the
various methodologies which can be used to evaluate health service
provision and an understanding of how the results from these can
be used to further develop performance management and quality
initiatives.

Summary

As this brief discussion has highlighted, quality of healthcare is a
complex matter. Perspectives on quality differ, and whilst a
common definition relating to the quality of NHS care has been
outlined in recent policy, this only places the onus on those
providing care to ensure that they are doing the right thing, at
the right time and in the right way. Achieving consensus between
all of the various interest groups about what is 'right' may take
some considerable time. Equally difficult is knowing where to focus
quality assessment programmes. Quality may be looked at in terms
of an organisation's structures, processes and outcomes, and
quality schemes will need to consider the inter-relationships
between the individual, group and organisation. Set against all of
these issues is the overarching question about *how* you assess
quality. It is to this topic that we now turn.

Chapter 3

Performance assessment

With the overriding concern to assure the quality of professional performance and to improve the quality of NHS care, developing and introducing review systems which adequately capture and reflect dimensions of individual and organisational performance has become a major area of professional, managerial, academic and political concern (Majeed and Voss 1995, Campbell *et al.* 1997, DoH 1998b, McColl *et al.* 1998, Giuffrida *et al.* 1999). This chapter briefly considers some of the quality and performance management initiatives of the past two decades which have left their legacy on today's NHS and then goes on to explore the various methodologies that can be employed for reviewing quality and performance. These include, for example, organisational accreditation schemes, national quality awards, professional quality programmes and benchmarking for primary care. The national framework for assessing performance is also outlined and its relevance for general practice discussed.

Key issues

The two major questions facing all those involved in the management and assessment of performance are:

1 how do you define what high-quality individual or organisational performance is?
2 how do you assess and develop this?

As the previous chapter highlighted, for those considering developing and implementing new quality schemes or performance review mechanisms there are a number of central themes which need to be considered. For example, when reviewing the quality of care provided by an organisation, what unit should form the basis for assessment? Is quality of service determined by what an individual clinician does, regardless of the outcome of such treatment or care? Conversely, should quality be seen in terms of health outcome measures – irrespective of how such outcomes are achieved? If quality is deemed to be a composite measure of what an individual practitioner does *and* the outcomes that are achieved, consideration needs to be given to the relationship between the two and how this might be assessed.

In looking at the outcomes of care, a number of different aspects can form the basis for assessment. Health gain, mortality and morbidity rates, appropriate treatment and patients' perceptions of health improvement could all be seen as salient outcome measures. Additionally, if performance is assessed in terms of outcomes it is also important to consider whether outcome is assessed at an individual patient level, by patient/population groups or in relation to the NHS or public sector as a whole (in reducing inequalities in health, for example). There are also broader economic measures which could apply to any assessment of performance (Drummond *et al.* 1987).

Equally, service providers do not work within a vacuum. The organisational infrastructure (e.g. systems, procedures, personnel and environment) and external factors (such as professional guidelines, policy initiatives, population characteristics) all impact on the ability of individual practitioners to provide appropriate care.

With clinical governance placing a statutory duty on all NHS organisations to monitor and improve the quality of service provision (however defined), performance management strategies will also have to consider how they advance the quality of care. This requires an understanding as to how and why poor performance occurs and also consideration about the interventions and resources required to improve the quality of care.

Building on the past

The recent initiatives which have sought to place quality at the heart of all NHS activities should not be seen in isolation. There has been a great deal of work undertaken in this field, and much of this provides valuable experience and information upon which to develop new performance management procedures.

> More work on quality has probably been done in the health care sector than in any other single public service. The literature is voluminous. It is also extremely varied, with a wide range of approaches and techniques being advocated. (CEPPP 1991)

It is important not to lose sight of the fact that:

> advancing quality in the UK means building on the legacy of the past, capitalising on existent knowledge, experience and technologies and integrating these with a new vision for the future of quality in the new NHS. (Leatherman and Sutherland 1998)

Key strategic developments include, for example:

- the introduction of general management into the NHS following the 1983 Griffiths Report
- the development of the NHS internal market, which sought to improve the efficiency, effectiveness, timeliness and quality of care through the separation of provider from purchaser – although a number of factors subsequently mitigated against this (Paton *et al.* 1998)
- *Health of the Nation* targets, which have been recently updated in *Our Healthier Nation* (DoH 1999b), identified particular disease groups in order to achieve improved health outcomes

- the *Patient's Charter* (DoH 1991) introduced the concept of performance targets for specific service areas and published league tables relating to performance

- a number of professionally orientated approaches seek to assess and develop the quality of professional practice (e.g. medical audit, critical incident reviews, the development of clinical guidelines and protocols, and the RCGP Membership and Fellowship by Assessment)

- national voluntary accreditation[1] programmes (e.g. King's Fund Primary Health Care Organisational Audit) which assess services according to a pre-determined set of standards

- from an organisational perspective, 'in-house' total quality management (TQM) and continuous quality improvement (CQI) schemes, business processing and re-engineering have all been used to develop local service provision. Additionally, a number of HAs have also introduced their own quality review schemes.

Despite the prevalence of a wide range of national and local initiatives to assess and develop the quality of NHS care, there are a number of unresolved issues. The piecemeal approach to assessing and developing service quality, for instance, is problematic. As several commentators have noted,

> *considerable resources are being directed at the process of monitoring, and as each authority undertakes this activity independently, each is finding different solutions. Not only does this consume . . . resources, it also defects the quest for equity in quality which might be expected within a national health service.* (Scrivens 1995)

However, not only do the methods used to assess performance

[1] 'Accreditation of health services organisations is concerned with assessing the quality of organisational processes and performance using agreed upon standards, compliance with which is assessed by surveyors' (Scrivens and Blaylock 1997)

differ, but the guidelines and standards against which services are assessed may themselves vary.

> Guidelines and standards have been formulated in a number of fields in the UK, but their development has been uneven. There is no organisation which has responsibility for standard setting across the board and the existence of standards in any particular field therefore depends upon the interests and inclinations of the bodies active in that field. (Ham and Hunter 1988)

Systems of review and standards for assessment

A range of review systems has been developed to assess the quality of NHS services. These systems can be organised in a number of ways, and may focus on the services provided by an organisation and/or an individual practitioner. As Scrivens (1995) notes,

> monitoring can be undertaken simply by the organisation for its own purposes, using its own assessment process. Alternatively, the measures of compliance may be borrowed from elsewhere but monitored by the organisation itself. A third possibility is that the organisation uses its own measures, but has them calibrated by a third party. A fourth is that the organisation uses measures from elsewhere which are also calibrated and checked by a third party.

This is shown diagrammatically in Figure 3.1.

Box 1 is the form of self-assessment which has traditionally been used by many organisations. Box 2 is a form of quality assurance which again many organisations have chosen to use in the past. Boxes 3 and 4 are forms of assessment which incorporate external measures – either in relation to the standards which are used or in relation to the process of validation. Box 4 is the normal type of accreditation activity in which external monitoring processes are imposed on the organisation.

Monitoring system		Assessment methods	
		Self	External
	Self	1 (i.e. HA in-house quality review scheme)	3
	External	2	4 (i.e. King's Fund Organisational Audit)

Figure 3.1   Monitoring/assessment matrix (Scrivens 1995).

In addition to the range of systems for monitoring and assessing quality, there are also a number of approaches to standard setting and monitoring compliance. With the new legislation aimed at ensuring a baseline quality of GP performance, many HAs are having to address what is meant by 'poor professional performance' and to develop standards, policies and procedures aimed at targeting those service providers whose performance gives cause for concern. Additionally, HAs are having to develop systems of review which not only monitor the provision of primary care services, but which are designed to promote quality practice. As we have seen, both of these approaches require consideration of the relationship between the performance of an individual, the context within which he or she works, the services which are provided and the outcomes of care (Gray 1992). As Chapter 2 has highlighted, any assessment might cover elements of:

- **structure** – which focuses on resources needed to support the actual provision of services (including equipment, personnel and facilities)

- **process** – which focuses on the activities which constitute the provision of services

- **outcomes** – which measure the consequences of management on a client's health status

- **professional aspects of service delivery** – these tend to be standards used to evaluate the professional activities or the technical nature of the service.

Historically, most quality assessment programmes have focused upon the nature of the organisation in which healthcare is delivered. Consequently, standards have typically concentrated on such things as the meeting of health and safety regulations, the correctness of administrative procedures, staffing and training policies, the existence of procedures and the processes used to create them – the assumption being that high-quality care cannot be provided if such factors are *not* in place. Outcome measures or the actual performance of an individual have not generally formed part of the assessment. More recently, quality programmes have sought to move away from a model which is primarily concerned with an assessment of structures and processes and have looked at ways to develop measures which assess *how well* an individual or organisation is performing. This moves us away from a concern with standards towards a model which has indicators against which performance can be assessed. Whilst standards and indicators are complementary, there are marked differences between them (*see* Box 3.1).

Indicators have been used in a variety of ways to assess the organisation and delivery of healthcare, and their different purposes tend to reflect the different organisational and political structures within which they have been developed.

In the USA, for example, performance indicators were originally developed in the accreditation systems to ensure that hospital organisations were provided in a manner which facilitated high-quality clinical care. They focused on aspects of organisational process and structure, and it is only recently that performance indicators have been developed which transcend organisational boundaries and look at care across a number of providers (i.e. a pathway/package of care). As with all healthcare systems, the need to provide some assessment of outcome is also having an impact on

---

Box 3.1: Standards and indicators

Standards are expectations or requirements for service provision. In the UK, for example, the King's Fund Organisational Audit had a range of standards used in assessments of primary care provision. These included:

Standards for primary health care team members

18.9 'There is evidence of on-going review of the audit cycle by the primary health care team'
18.10 'Confidentiality is maintained throughout the evaluation process'
18.11 'Staff participate in the formulation of plans for improvement'
                    King's Fund Organisational Audit Primary Health Care
                    Organisational Standards and Criteria (1996 Manual)

Standards which merely denote whether a particular feature is in place have been developed further in the USA. As Gilpatrick (1999) observes:

> *In the USA, the Joint Commission for Accreditation of Healthcare Organisations standards purport to define the structures, functions and processes needed to achieve good patient outcomes. They not only name the processes or functions, but [have been developed to] include threshold criteria or limits for what acceptable performance is.*

By contrast, **an indicator** is:

• a quantifiable measure that can be used as a guide to monitor and evaluate the quality of important patient care and support activities (JCAHO 1989)

• a valid and reliable quantitative process or outcome measure related to one or more dimensions of performance, such as effectiveness and appropriateness, and a statistical value that provides an indication of the condition or direction over time of an organisation's performance of a specified outcome (JCAHO 1995).

> *An indicator might measure patient's length of stay, no. of falls per 1000 days, the % of patients waiting for a procedure beyond an acceptable period, % of deliveries by caesarian section or the number of deaths within a certain time period after a surgical procedure. Generally expressed as a rate, ratio or percentage, an indicator can be compared from one organisation to another. When compared with established criteria an indicator can identify areas that are not doing well and warrant more detailed analysis. Although indicators report on past performance, they can trigger exploration of causes which, when found, can result in system changes that are likely to improve future care.* (Gilpatrick 1999)

the nature of the performance indicators which are being developed (JCAHO 1995, Scrivens and Blaylock 1997).

In the USA, the incentive to undertake some form of organisational quality assessment came with the introduction of Medicare and Medicaid. 'This, in effect, made hospitals dependent upon revenue from tax-financed patients. Public finance brought about a threat of public regulation: the reimbursement of Medicare patients was made dependent on hospitals meeting the federal conditions, enforced by states, for participation' (Scrivens 1995). In 42 states in the USA, those hospitals who successfully participate in the JCAHO accreditation programme are, by virtue of adhering to national standards and indicators for healthcare delivery, deemed to have met the conditions for participation in Medicare and are therefore exempt from state regulatory processes. The whole question of developing, implementing and meeting indicators has therefore become an integral part of healthcare provision in these systems.

In the UK, with different service configurations, professional structures and methods of financing healthcare, indicators have not developed in a similar format. Whilst considerable attention has been given to key areas of health service activity (e.g. finished consultant episodes, waiting lists, league tables) such indicators do not focus on the organisation of care nor do they consider how care is delivered (and indeed some of these may be thought of in terms of out*puts* as opposed to out*comes*).

In terms of how standards and indicators are developed and monitored there are several different approaches which may be combined in a number of ways as shown in Figure 3.2. Box 1 suggests a host of locally dominated systems run by many possible organisations. Box 2 suggests nationally agreed standards (and/or indicators) which are then implemented locally, which may generate statistical returns for comparisons to be made by, for example, the Department of Health (or national quality schemes). Box 3 is a highly flexible system allowing for local variations in service provision to be taken into account but with some national

Monitoring system		Standards' development	
		Local	National
	Local	1	2
	National	3	4

Figure 3.2   Monitoring/standards matrix.

system checking the implementation of standards. Box 4 suggests a national accreditation system of the kind found in the USA, Canada or Australia (Scrivens 1995).

There are:

> *different and totally unrelated arguments as to how standards should be set and how the process of monitoring should be conducted. There are a number of different foci for the systems of standard setting which relate to whether quality is to be assessed in the process or in the outcome. This in turn affects the decision as to whether the assessment is better undertaken internally by the organisation itself or externally by an outside body. If quality is to be assessed in the process then standards will relate to definitions of good practice and will attempt to control how health care is delivered. This requires therefore, an externally agreed definition of process to which all parties subscribe. However, if the processes for achieving quality are felt to be best left to internal management, then quality will tend to be assessed using measures which either attempt to impose some measurement of quality assurance processes or to examine the outcome of the process. (Scrivens 1995)*

> **Key issues**
> - Who controls the processes of standard setting and monitoring?
> - To what extent should this be internal or external to the organisation?

Where to focus attention

Given that much recent attention has been focused on the question of reducing variations in the quality of NHS care (DoH 1997), it may well be the case that the overriding concern of HAs, PCGs and local medical committees is to ensure that all GP-based services are provided to an acceptable level. Under such circumstances, it is possible that relatively little attention is given to those individuals or groups who provide care deemed to be well above any minimum agreed standard. Whilst minimum standards for service provision seek to ensure a *baseline* quality of service provision – 'levels below which any operation would be unacceptable' (Scrivens 1995) – such standards do not necessarily reflect what are thought to be the *optimum* or the highest achievable standards. There may be significant differences therefore between those schemes which are designed to ensure a minimum standard of service provision and those which promote quality development through the use of 'gold' standards. The different emphasis impacts on the nature of the standards and indicators used.

With publication of *The New NHS: Modern and Dependable – A National Framework for Assessing Performance* (DoH 1998b) greater standardisation is advocated in the quality assessment process. Key areas of service provision have been outlined so that performance can be assessed according to various dimensions (e.g. by population group, by disease, by HA or trust, by service/sector) and a small number of outcome-based performance indicators will provide national and local information about the provision of services. These are designed 'to help managers and clinicians to work together to review their performance and improve the quality, effectiveness and efficiency and outcomes of the services they provide [through] greater benchmarking of performance in different areas and the publication of comparative information' (DoH 1998b, p. 6). It is envisaged that these national performance indicators will sit alongside other techniques for assessing the quality of services.

The government therefore has shied away from developing a rigorous and *comprehensive* national performance review structure and has opted instead for establishing new bodies for overseeing quality and performance within the NHS (NICE and CHI), for implementing an overarching performance framework and for promoting *local* clinical governance.

National performance indicators

Although the use of standards and indicators against which to assess performance is something of a 'contested terrain' (Majeed and Voss 1995, Campbell *et al.* 1997, DoH 1998a, McColl *et al.* 1998, Giuffrida *et al.* 1999), performance indicators are well developed in the established accreditation systems of Canada, the USA and Australia. Whilst their introduction into the NHS arena does not follow a similar developmental path and there is widespread debate about the validity, reliability and sensitivity of indicators to assess individual and organisational performance, the inclusion of performance indicators in the new national framework signals that, if appropriately developed and used, they are regarded centrally as suitable methods of assessing performance.

> *Setting standards, delivering standards, monitoring standards – these are the routes to consistent, prompt, high quality services throughout the NHS . . . For the first time in the history of the NHS standards will be set for how services should be delivered.*

The Government, the NHS and the public need to know whether services really are delivering the high quality care that patients have a right to expect. (DoH 1998a)

The latest White Paper and consultation papers on a national framework for assessing performance outline a number of indicators for both acute and primary care services. These are designed to provide comparative information about the quality of NHS care in several key areas. This parallels moves in other countries including Scotland, where performance indicator measures (focused on outcomes) have been made public for a number of years. The national framework marks the 'start of a process which will lead over time to a comprehensive assessment of those aspects of performance which really matter. It will encourage greater benchmarking of performance in different areas and the publication of comparative information will allow people to compare performance and share best practice' (DoH 1998b).

The national framework focuses on six key areas, and each one has a number of potential indicators for assessing provision as outlined in Table 3.1.

It is anticipated that 'high level' indicators will:

provide an overview of NHS performance to inform the performance management process, encourage national and local improvements in performance and support public accountability. However, there will clearly be other issues not captured . . . where there will be a need for effective performance management to achieve improvements in health and health care. (DoH 1997)

The national performance indicators consist in the main of:

• **composite indicators** (combining several sets of data to give an overall picture) and

• **sentinel indicators** (single indicators which reflect performance in a wider area).

Table 3.1   Key areas of policy and potential indicators

Area	Potential indicators
Health improvement	• Public health common data set • *Our Healthier Nation* Green Paper indicators • Standardised mortality ratios • Health expectancy
Fair access	• Variations in the take up of services, as shown by other indicators, give information on equity of access
Effective delivery of appropriate healthcare	• Community care • Prescribing • Clinical effectiveness indicators • Primary care effectiveness indicators • Mental health • Continuing care
Efficiency	• Unit costs/labour productivity index • Capital productivity/costed HRGs
Patient/carer experience	• Waiting times /Patient's Charter/NHS Charter • National survey on patient/carer experiences
Health outcomes of NHS care	• Population health outcomes/mental health • Outcomes

Compositing allows the set of indicators to remain relatively small in number whilst still encompassing a wide range of aspects of NHS performance. This approach is:

> analogous to the Retail Price Index, where price movements of numerous different items are weighted and summarised in a single high level measure. Such an approach provides an additional, summary, level of information for particular areas for use within the . . . framework whilst the individual constituent indicators, within a composite measure, are available from their original sources to enable more in-depth analysis as appropriate. (DoH 1998b)

Alongside this overall framework, there are specific areas which have been developed in more detail, including clinical effectiveness indicators.

The national clinical effectiveness indicators

The clinical effectiveness indicators consultation document:

> *sets out the initial results of a work programme to develop national comparative indicators of clinical effectiveness and describes how they link with the new national performance framework and the clinical effectiveness performance development framework . . . Although useful in themselves as a stand alone tool, they are also an integral part of the revised approach to assessing and developing NHS performance.* (DoH 1998c)

It is envisaged that the introduction of these indicators will assist HAs in the monitoring of performance, since they:

> *will provide useful benchmarking information which should complement other, more detailed, local information and be of interest to individual clinicians.*

The proposed national clinical effectiveness indicators relate to 14 population-based rates of healthcare interventions, covering both hospital and non-hospital based care. Each indicator was carefully selected on the basis of evidence and other factors which suggested one of the following.

- There is an unmet need for effective intervention and a high rate would be desirable.

- A number of patients are receiving the intervention inappropriately and a decreasing rate would be desirable.

- There is variation in the rate of effective intervention but it is currently unclear whether a higher or lower rate would be desirable.

The documentation published by the NHS Executive includes a chart for each indicator, illustrating the latest HA data from HAs, grouped by the relevant year. Those indicators which fall into the first two categories outlined above include a suggested national change of direction. Accompanying each indicator is a detailed description of:

- the indicator

- the purpose of the intervention

- the rationale for the indicator

- factors to consider when interpreting it

- references and a list of other complimentary 'effectiveness products'.

The indicators are loosely based around the following categories of:

- health promotion/disease prevention

- early detection

- diagnostic assessment/investigation

- treatment/rehabilitation care

- long-term care/support

Selection of the national clinical effectiveness indicators

The national clinical effectiveness indicators were developed by a working group representing a broad range of stakeholders such as clinical practitioners, clinical effectiveness experts and researchers. The group's objective was to agree a 'basket' of clinical indicators for consultation, based on existing evidence. A number of criteria for selection were drawn up and the working group commissioned the Health Services Management Centre in Birmingham to review each potential indicator against the criteria and to hold discussions with a small number of clinical practitioners. The results from this process were used in determining which indicators should be included in the overall clinical effectiveness framework. Over time it is envisaged that further indicators may be added to the clinical effectiveness indicator set, dependent upon such factors as improved data collection or the results of research. The 14 indicators were selected because of their focus on important service issues where, in general, the evidence is well established and routine data are available. The problems in data collection meant that other indicators which were deemed suitable for inclusion, could not be established within a national programme.

> *The 14 proposed indicators should not be interpreted as priorities for clinical effectiveness to the exclusion of other interventions and services, or to the reduction in promoting the other four strands of the integrated approach set out in the Clinical Effectiveness Performance Development Framework.* (DoH 1998c)

During 1998 widespread consultation took place regarding these indicators and they were 'road tested' throughout the country on a regional basis. It is envisaged that, in due course, the indicator set will be of relevance to:

- the public, patients and their representatives
- service providers
- HAs and PCGs
- ministers and the NHS Executive.

Limitations of the national clinical effectiveness indicators

Several caveats to the clinical effectiveness indicators are detailed in the official documentation. These include how variations might occur and how health professionals might address such issues, whether any inappropriate interventions occur and also suggesting a national change of direction. Technical information on data sources, data quality, robustness of data, confidence intervals, clustering, data years and standardisation was also included in the consultation document (DoH 1998c). It was also felt to be essential that the clinical effectiveness indicators were used in concert with other national and local indicators and should complement routine quality improvement tools such as clinical audit and clinical guidelines.

Data sources

Whilst the new framework for assessing performance highlights the move towards specific measures of performance, the difficulties of collating and analysing data remain a major barrier to further indicator development. As the White Paper acknowledges,

> *to avoid additional burdens of the NHS from new data collection, and to enable early progress to be made, the indicator set will initially make use of information that is already available at HA level. This will mean in particular that some of the high level indicators are far from ideal and that some of them will use process measures as a proxy for information that is not yet available on outcomes, effectiveness and quality. The high level indicator set will be developed over time as better, more outcomes focused data becomes available. But it is intended that the set will remain small . . . The small set of indicators is not intended to be comprehensive in covering all aspects of NHS activities. However, so far as data availability allows, the indicators have been chosen to throw light on particularly important health service objectives and activities.*

The national framework and general practice

The indicators proposed in the national framework for assessing performance that are most relevant to primary care and cited by McColl *et al.* (1998) are shown in Box 3.2.

Box 3.2: The national framework and general practice

Fair access

- To elective surgery: rates of CABG* and PTCA**, of hip and knee replacement and of cataract replacement.

- To family planning services: conception rates for those aged <16.

- To cancer screening services: % of target population screened for breast and cervical cancer.

- To district nurse contacts: district nurse and assistant district nurse contacts for those aged >75 and district nurse contacts lasting >30 minutes for the same age group.

Effective delivery of healthcare

- % of target population vaccinated and % of all orchidopexies for those aged <5.

- % of target population screened for breast and cervical cancer (as above).

- Rates of CABG and PTCA, of hip and knee replacement and of cataract replacement.

- Age and sex standardised admission rates for severe ENT infection, kidney and urinary tract infection, heart failure ('avoidable admissions').

- Age and sex standardised admission rates for asthma, diabetes and epilepsy ('largely managed in primary care').

- Volume of prescribing of benzodiazepines and ratio of antidepressants to benzodiazepines.

- Composite measure of prescribing of combination and modified release products plus drugs of limited clinical value and inhaled corticosteroids.

Efficiency

- % generic prescribing.

---

*   CABG = coronary artery bypass graft
** PTCA = percutaneous transluminal coronary angioplasty

Box 3.3: Health outcomes of NHS care

• Conception rates for those aged <16.

• Notification rates for pertussis and measles.

• Emergency hospital admissions for people aged >75.

• Rates of emergency psychiatric readmission.

And the *Clinical Effectiveness Indicators* consultation document (1998) also proposes several key indicators which directly reflect the performance of general practice (*see* Table 3.2).

Table 3.2 Key clinical effectiveness indicators for general practice

Area	Clinical effectiveness indicator	
Health promotion/ disease prevention	1	Prescribing rate of statins in general practice
	2	Childhood immunisation for MMR in England 1996/7
Early detection	3 & 4	Cervical/breast cancer screening
Treatment/rehabilitation care	10	Prescribing rate of benzodiazepines in general practice
	12	CABG/PTCA rates

Each indicator is presented in the manner shown in Table 3.3.

What we see therefore, with the new framework document and the development of national, evidence-based indicators for particular areas of service provision, is a move towards some form of comparative and standardised assessment of NHS performance. However, with the advent of clinical governance, all NHS organisations will have to demonstrate that they are continuously monitoring and reviewing performance in *all* areas. This latter requirement demands some form of local or organisational-specific strategy. Equally, not only will NHS organisations have to monitor

Table 3.3   CEI 2: Childhood immunisation for MMR in England 1996/7

Indicator definition	The percentage of children immunised with MMR by their second birthday. The HAs should aim to immunise 95% of the target population.
Numerator	The number of children resident in the HA at 31 March who reached their second birthday in the preceding year and who are recorded as having had an MMR vaccination before their second birthday.
Area	Health promotion/disease prevention.
Rationale for indicator	There is strong evidence of clinical effectiveness for childhood immunisation programmes and this is a robust indicator which is currently in use. The aim should be to achieve as near to 100% uptake as possible and there is still considerable scope for raising rates to ensure uniformly high uptake. This indicator shows the extent of variation across the country and that the majority of districts still need to increase uptake levels to reach the 95% target.
Purpose of intervention	Primary prevention and production of herd immunity to measles, mumps and rubella. Measles is a highly infectious viral illness with complication in 1 in 15 cases, hospitalisation in 1 in 100 cases, meningitis/encephalitis in 1 in 1000 cases and death in 1 in 2500 to 5000 cases. Mumps is an acute viral illness of varying severity, characterised by swelling of one or both parotid salivary glands; complications include pancreatitis, meningo-encephalitis, oophoritis and orchitis. Rubella is a mild or subacute viral illness. Although rarely serious for the sufferer, there can be serious ill effects from maternal rubella infection. Rubella in the first 8–10 weeks of pregnancy results in fetal damage in up to 90% of infants and multiple defects are common.
Data	Cover of Vaccination Evaluated Rapidly (COVER) returns made to the Communicable Disease Surveillance Centre (CDSC).
Interpretation of indicator	• Special features – The intervention (of measles immunisation) is about 90–95% effective. Mathematical modelling predicts that 95% uptake is needed at both of the immunisation time points (primary and pre-school) to eradicate measles. This should be the case even if it is the same 95% who are immunised each time.

Table 3.3   (*cont.*)

	• Information issues – inadequate child health information systems, GPs failing to send returns to the local child health computer promptly or at all and miscoding will influence accuracy of data. • A low rate of MMR uptake might indicate any of the influences listed below.
Likely influences on the rate of intervention	• Social (lower rates related to deprivation, lone parenthood, large family size). • Cultural and media (influencing parental beliefs about both the value and complications of the intervention, availability of childcare). • Structural (e.g. accessibility of service). • Mobility of resident population. • Educational (information and enthusiasm imparted by health professionals). True contraindications exist in fewer than 1% of children. While immunisation is strongly encouraged, participation remains voluntary and parents exercise choice as to whether or not children are immunised.
Question for consultation	Childhood immunisation covers a range of vaccines. Is MMR the most useful to highlight for this indicator or should another aspect of the childhood immunisation programme be identified? Should DTP and polio be included?

their performance, but they will also have to demonstrate that the measures that they introduce to achieve such aims are themselves robust. For those wishing to develop their quality review mechanisms, it may be worthwhile looking at pre-existing quality review schemes as well as initiating 'in-house' systems for performance assessment.

Where do we start and what do we do?

There are a range of schemes and techniques which have been developed to assess the quality of both organisational and individual practice. Some of these have a national focus, with common standards and criteria applicable to all organisations, others look for a more locally orientated approach to performance assessment and quality improvement. Both have their value, and with clinical governance requiring all NHS organisations to develop an over-arching and integrated approach to performance management, new ways of thinking about quality improvement and performance management may be needed. Developing and implementing effective clinical governance is made more difficult by the fact that varying approaches will have to be used to ensure appropriate performance management. Ensuring that the correct organisational structures, policies and procedures are in place, for example, will require a very different currency from systems which review professional competencies. The art of developing clinical govern-ance lies in understanding what each technique, programme or methodology has to offer, and how this might fit within an organisation's overall approach to clinical governance.

The following section briefly reviews a range of national or comparative approaches which has been developed to assess organisational and personal performance.

• Accreditation and organisational audit schemes

• RCGP programmes to assess the quality of general practice (individual and collective)

• ISO 9000

• 'Charter Mark'

• Benchmarking

• 'Investors in People'

• Clinical audit

In addition to these programmes, there are also broader approaches to monitoring and developing quality of care. Total quality management and continuous quality improvement repres-ent two of these, and they are discussed briefly here.

Accreditation schemes

Accreditation in healthcare is a means of reviewing the
quality of the organisation of healthcare using external
surveyors and published standards (Scrivens 1995).
It should not be confused with the accreditation of
practices/organisations for professional training purposes,
nor should it be taken to encompass professional
're-accreditation' or 're-certification' whereby the
competency of individuals to practice is assessed.

A number of organisations have looked towards the established
hospital accreditation schemes as an appropriate model for developing quality review schemes for primary or practice-based care.
The original accreditation programmes, developed in the USA,
Canada and Australia, focused on the provision of hospital-based
services and were founded on the premise that there are certain
actions and characteristics which should be in place to create a
good service (for a detailed account *see* Scrivens 1995).

Every accreditation programme employs a system or process for
measuring the organisation or the service against specific standards. This process involves determination of the standards and the
processes (if used) for 'scoring' the performance of the organisation
or ranking it against others. Hospital accreditation programmes
typically assess the quality of organisational processes and performance against selected criteria, using external surveyors. Participation in accreditation programmes is usually voluntary and results
in the award of a grading or 'score' which denotes the degree of
compliance with the standards.

The purpose of the original accreditation programmes was to
establish and encourage best practice in the control of hospital
management systems. Although the scope of hospital programmes
has expanded, the basic premise – that there are certain actions

which should be undertaken to create a 'good hospital' and that the prime concern should be with the protection of staff and patients – has remained unchanged. This form of organisational accreditation is distinct from professional 'accreditation', the latter of which is used to approve facilities for professional training purposes (although there may be some overlap between those aspects of care which form the basis of assessment).

Despite cultural differences in the practice of healthcare, hospitals are remarkably similar institutions. However, within primary and community care there is often a distinct lack of any common organisation or structure and the services provided vary considerably – both by location and by provider. As services outside hospitals tend to be provided by a variety of different organisations, a single patient may be the recipient of care from a number of different providers who may themselves be employed by different organisations (Scrivens and Blaylock 1997). This has major implications for the development of quality assurance programmes which seek to assess the quality of such care. Whilst a number of accreditation systems have been attempting to find ways of linking the accreditation process across different services – the Commission on Accreditation of Rehabilitation Facilities (CARF) in the USA, for example, is a traditional accreditation system which was developed to cut across organisational boundaries, and in the UK Health Services Accreditation has emphasised the needs of patients attending A&E departments – the emphasis of the majority of accreditation programmes has remained focused on organisational structures and processes. As Scrivens and Blaylock (1997) note:

> . . . the success of hospital accreditation systems lies in the consensus achieved across the many professions which contribute to the working of a hospital about the standards to define its work. There is no such consensus in primary and community care services which means that any search for consensus has to recognise the variation in the organisation of services.

This problem is not unique to the UK, as the development of accreditation programmes in Australia has highlighted.

> The complexity and diversity and multi-disciplinary nature of community health services in Australia means that developing standards is a challenging task . . . such standards must be specific enough to be usable and capable of being evaluated once they are applied but broad enough to cover diverse local circumstances. (Fry 1990)

When moving outside the acute sector, the traditional approach to accreditation has been followed, with the emphasis still placed on structures and processes. This has resulted in a search for organisational structures which can form the basis for an accreditation approach. As a result, many non-acute schemes use the general practice as the focus for assessment, as the following two examples illustrate.

King's Fund 'Health Quality Service' Award

The King's Fund is an independent charity in the UK which promotes good practice and improvement in health and social care through grants, information, services and management development, policy analysis and audit. The original King's Fund Organisational Audit (KFOA) for primary care was an independent and voluntary audit of the whole practice using a set of standards and criteria, developed by the King's Fund for use throughout the country. The standards and criteria:

> relate to the systems and processes required to support the delivery of primary health care service. The audit involves the evaluation of compliance with these standards by means of an external peer review . . . the KFOA sets out to complement local and professional initiatives, recognise and spread good practice and support continuous organisational development. (King's Fund 1996)

The standards against which services are assessed are continually being reviewed and were:

> *designed for the providers of those services – GPs and members of the primary health care team. The standards can help them to develop the organisations in which they work (and the way they commission services) systematically and consistently over time.*

The standards and criteria relate to a number of different areas of provision:

- Patient's/client's rights
- Policies, procedures and protocols
- Service level agreements
- Patient/client access to services
- Management of commissioning
- Management of medicines
- Communication and team working
- Health record system
- Information
- Strategy and objectives
- Health and safety
- Management arrangements
- Patient/client care
- Staff development and education
- Health record content
- Referrals and investigations
- Buildings/facilities and equipment

and were developed to be:

- Measurable – both by the staff implementing the criteria and by the surveyors assessing compliance against them.

- Achievable – some organisations will find it more difficult to achieve the criteria than others, but there is little point in including criteria that are not achievable.

- Flexible – so they can be used by any primary healthcare team.

- Acceptable – representing a consensus on currently accepted roles and responsibilities.

- Adaptable – non-prescriptive (stating what should be in place and not how it should be in place) so they can be implemented in accordance with local needs.

- Nationally applicable – a common framework against which all primary healthcare teams within the UK can be assessed.

Box 3.4: An example of KFOA standards

Under policies, procedures and protocols:

• Written policies are developed by the primary healthcare team.

• Written policies are shared with the primary healthcare team (essential practice) and patients (good practice).

• When writing policies, the relevant influences, such as statutory regulations, codes of ethics and local/national agreed objectives are considered.

The cost of going through the KFOA was £6000 per practice, and practices have often received support from their HA in order to undertake this form of external assessment.

The RCGP Organisational Accreditation Programme

The RCGP has sought to develop accreditation for primary health care *teams* on the basis that:

• the underlying ethos of accreditation should be to support quality improvement in practice and to be closely related to practice development and education

• it is not the concern of the practice accreditation programme to assess the performance of the individual doctor (since this should be part of a process of re-certification); accreditation should be concerned with the practice team and its functioning and the services the team provides

• because the RCGP is concerned with the work of the primary care team, both the setting of the criteria and the assessment should be multidisciplinary.

Initially it was envisaged that any method of practice accreditation should be voluntary, but designed so that every practice could participate. The RCGP promotes voluntary participation in such schemes on the basis that 'a good voluntary system is better than a compulsory one which encourages compliance with minimal standards rather than striving for optimal standards' (RCGP 1996, personal interview). It was also proposed that the assessment methods should build on existing methods of review conducted by the team, such as clinical audit, quality improvement initiatives and surveys of the views of patients. This model of practice accreditation is still in its infancy, with a pilot scheme having been undertaken in Brent and Harrow (the principles of which are as follows).

RCGP practice accreditation programme
Content and criteria for assessment

- Both the setting of criteria and the assessment should be multidisciplinary.

- The criteria should reflect the needs of patients.

- The criteria should cover the range of services that can be provided by practices.

- Criteria for individuals in the team should relate to their training and certification.

- Levels of performance should not just define minimum standards but indicate markers to encourage progress in practice. They should be described as essential, normal, good practice and desirable.

- Essential criteria should be those that relate to terms and conditions of service, professional requirements, legal requirements or safety of practice.

- Wherever possible, criteria should not just reflect professional or patient opinion, but also evidence of relationship to outcomes.

Methods of assessment

- Assessment should be by peers and therefore multidisciplinary.

- Assessment methods should build upon existing methods of review.

- Practice visiting should be used to validate the self-assessment, assess those features which cannot be assessed in other ways and to establish a relationship for constructive feedback.

- The method of assessment must be demonstrably valid and reliable.

Responsibility

- Local steering groups should include representatives of professional bodies, HAs and patients.

- Local steering groups should have strong links with professional educational bodies.

The scheme has been evaluated by the HSMC, Birmingham. Piloting revealed that the consequences for poor performance have yet to be fully addressed. The Working Party document notes that 'initially, accreditation will be a pilot project, but consideration should be given now to the implications of PHCTs failing to reach minimum standards. We recommend that this should lead to remedial action and not to sanctions'.

The RCGP Quality Practice Award

In addition to developing a practice-based accreditation pro-gramme, the RCGP has already developed a Quality Practice Award (QPA) to provide a national quality scheme for practices. The scheme requires a high level of performance, somewhere between the standards required for Fellowship by Assessment and Membership by Assessment of Performance. The award was set up in 1995 under the guidance of the Quality Practice Award Working Party and was piloted in the North East Scotland Faculty of the RCGP in 1996 with the help of a grant from the Primary Care Development Fund.

The QPA works by focusing on the key functions of general practice and also reflects the patients' perspective by asking what they would expect of a practice which has achieved such an award. All practices applying for the QPA are required to meet set criteria ranging from demonstrating details of clinical care to health and safety issues, all of which must be submitted in the form of written evidence. The criteria are regularly modified and developed to reflect ongoing changes in general practice.

Once a practice's application has been submitted and reviewed, preparations are made for a spot check and a day-long visit to the practice during which the assessment team will interview staff and patients and inspect the premises. The QPA focuses on all members of the PCT and the assessors are also multidisciplinary. The award is granted for five years, and any practice can apply, whether or not the doctors are members of the RCGP. Established in 1997, 50 practices are currently working towards QPA, with four practices having been awarded QPA recognition and three awaiting assessment (summer 1999 figures).

One of the major problems in using accreditation-type schemes is that accreditation (or similar external organisational audit programmes) only show what an organisation is *capable* of doing. Whilst ensuring that good practice management is in place and that the organisation has clear and sound methods of working, most programmes tend to focus on how care is organised (i.e. reviewing aspects of structure and process) as opposed to how care is delivered (from practitioner to patient) or looking at the outcomes of care. One of the key challenges facing PCGs and PCTs is to deliver measurable improvements to the health of their practice population. For those charged with leading the clinical governance agenda it will therefore be necessary to develop and implement performance management programmes which also look at the *impact* that services have on particular patient and population groups.

Training practices

As we have seen in Chapter 2, individual GPs may apply to become trainers, and their practices are accredited as training practices. Accreditation involves assessment of both the doctor (e.g. commitment to audit and personal professional development) and the practice (e.g. good premises, high standards of records).

ISO 9000 (formerly BS 5750)

This quality award focuses on sets of procedures to ensure accountability and the systematic review of services provided by an organisation. It is not specifically related to healthcare but is applicable to any organisation wishing to undertake a review of their internal procedures. It is particularly relevant in the current health policy climate given that it also reviews systems which facilitate feedback from users. Compliance with national standards is assessed during a two-day visit by British Standards Institute (BSI) inspectors. The fee for a small practice is approximately £3500, followed by £1600 annual registration.

Charter Mark

The Charter Mark scheme recognises commitment to quality practice throughout the public sector. For those practices who wish to apply for a Charter Mark, clear evidence of improvements in quality of a service across a range of topics has to be submitted. At the same time, practices have to demonstrate that they are continually striving to improve the quality of their services through innovative working practices. Whilst the Charter Mark is a nationally recognised award, there are no uniform standards and criteria; organisations who seek to be awarded Charter Mark status develop their own criteria and use self-assessment as a means to demonstrate the quality of their service. For those awarded Charter Mark status, evidence must be submitted every three years to keep the Charter Mark. There is no on-site inspection or fee involved in the Charter Mark scheme.

The Charter Mark, whilst indicating a clear commitment to quality within any public sector organisation, does not signify equity between organisations in their quality, achievements and practices and Charter Marks may be stripped from those organisations who fail to demonstrate quality in their service, as the case of the Passport Office in 1999 illustrates.

Benchmarking

In 1996 the NHS Benchmarking Club was established to encourage the use of benchmarking, a management tool for the comparative assessment of NHS organisations. The club, which currently comprises 40 HAs, 100 PCGs, and 8 associate members (Audit Commission, Department of Health, Welsh Office, 4 regional offices and a FHSA), has recently completed the first stage of a project designed to benchmark the state of primary care. Using data from 23 HAs and 2270 practices the project revealed considerable variations across a range of indicators throughout England and Wales (Rodger and Watkins 1999). Some of the key indicators included

- % of practices achieving 60% generic prescribing
- % of inadequate smears
- % of practices with pathology links
- breast cancer screening coverage rates
- % of practices linked to the NHS net
- % of practices with a business plan.

The project is on-going and further indicators are being developed to reflect the changing nature of primary care. Whilst the findings undoubtedly enable those HAs where provision falls short of an agreed benchmark to go back and review local provision, disaggregation of some of the practice-level data is required if one is to assess provision at an individual practitioner level.

In addition, NHS Estates (part of the NHS Executive) have introduced a patient questionnaire which looks at users' experiences across a range of aspects of service provision. These are predominantly focused on hospital-based care and include access availability, reception/waiting area, general surroundings and confidentiality. There are fewer questions concerning general practice care. For those who wish to gauge the response of users to local services, this scheme provides a useful method and one which can be implemented at relatively little cost. For a fee of £350, the NHS Estates provide the questionnaire and will also undertake analysis and feedback. Given the standardised format this approach also facilitates inter-organisational comparisons. However, because the questionnaire is not specifically orientated towards general practice, a more focused primary care-based research tool is required to assess users' perceptions of the quality of general practice.

Investors in People

With recent initiatives such as *Working Together* and clinical governance (and the associated human resource management implications), Investors in People provides a valuable point of reference for those wishing to demonstrate their organisation's commitment to 'valuing staff through good practice, training and development'. However, this scheme is not specific to health service organisations and there may be aspects of professional medical practice, regulation and development which need special consideration. Under the scheme, a catalogue of evidence is prepared, followed by an inspection by two assessors. The cost of participating in the scheme is approximately £1000.

Fellowship and Membership of the RCGP

Fellowship and Membership of the RCGP have already been discussed in the context of professional views about the constituent components of high-quality care within general practice. Nonetheless, it is worth recapping the major points in order that they can be compared to other external quality schemes. The Membership by Assessment and Fellowship by Assessment are particularly relevant since they focus on aspects of individual practice as well as considering the context within which care is delivered.

The RCGP operates a scheme whereby members of the College may become Fellows by assessment. This contrasts with the more traditional scheme of peer 'nomination' to the position of Fellow. The assessment process involves 'detailed preparation by the doctor, which includes standards of records, personnel issues and clinical audits and which typically lasts between one and three years. Inspection by a visiting team includes assessment of a videotape of the doctor's consultations' (Roland *et al.* 1998). Although this form of assessment captures the range of inter-personal and organisational factors which contribute to practice-based care, only a relatively small number of individuals have gone through this process. By the end of 1998, for example, only approximately 150 doctors had achieved Fellowship by Assessment.

Within the UK, roughly half of all GPs have taken the Member-ship of the RCGP examination. This seeks to promote high standards throughout general practice. In 1999, in common with the shifting emphasis towards direct assessment of professional competencies *in situ*, Membership by Assessment of Performance was introduced, providing an alternative route of entry to the College for established GPs who have not taken the RCGP membership exam.

Clinical audit

Clinical audit (together with education, training and professional self-regulation) is the mainstay of ensuring quality in professional practice. In 1986, the RCGP policy statement on quality in general practice recommended that clinical audit should be developed within all practices and should be seen not only as an educational tool for practitioners, but also as an aid to assessing the manage-ment of the whole practice. Medical audit throughout the NHS was introduced under the Thatcher government and Medical Audit Advisory Groups (MAAGs) were subsequently introduced by the

Department of Health in order to promote and develop audit in all general practices. Today, the scope of audit in general practice encompasses not only the activities of medical practitioners, but also the performance of the practice team and the interface between general practice and other providers. However, whilst many practices undertake audit on a regular basis, in general practice (unlike in the acute sector) audit remains voluntary and, as with other aspects of innovation or change, it is often left to key individuals to champion its development.

A useful summary of the purposes and methods of audit is provided by Irvine and Irvine (1996). In addition to the external purposes of audit (i.e. for 'external comparison and review') they regard audit as being central to internal performance monitoring.

'Internal clinical audit has five functions in particular:

- Monitoring compliance with guidelines, both clinical and operational – are we doing what we said we would?

- Minimising risk, by helping to reduce clinical and organisational error

- As an aid to learning, by showing gaps in skills and knowledge

- As an way of helping to bring about change by documenting the progress of change

- In reducing frustration by showing why maddening things actually happen – regularly lost case notes for example

and may be carried out by a variety of methods:

- Routine performance monitoring

- Practice activity analysis

- Surveys and interviews

- Direct observation

- Significant event analysis

- Use of tracers.'

With the move towards evidenced-based practice throughout the whole of the NHS and with the establishment of the NICE and clinical governance, the place of audit within general practice must assume higher significance. Audit serves as a monitoring, evaluative and educational tool and can also focus on the activities of individuals, teams and organisations (and the relationships between these) as well as considering the package of care provided to individual patients or patient/disease groups (*see* Figure 3.3).

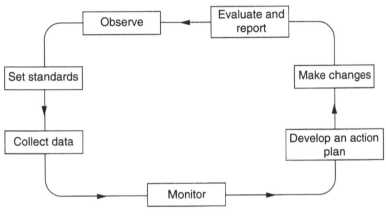

Figure 3.3   Audit cycle.

One of the major barriers to further development of audit in general practice was alluded to in the recent framework document for assessing performance – that of the seemingly ever-present problem in the NHS of data (availability, accuracy, reliability, validity, etc.). However, with the need for systems which demonstrate a commitment to strong performance management, all providers and commissioners will have to promote mechanisms which safeguard and improve standards of care. For this organisations should consider not only the data that they currently collect and analyse, but also consider what data will be required to meet future requirements. 'Good data provides the basis for the comparative analyses from which it is possible to see the actual performance in relation to pre-set standards and also to identify

patterns that may provide the starting point for further enquiries'
(Irvine and Irvine 1996). It is also worthwhile noting that outcomes
(i.e. the impact of care) will play an increasing role in performance
management programmes. Although limited outcome data have
been looked at within clinical audit (e.g. mortality, adverse
incidents, prescribing data), assessments of the outcomes of care
provided by an individual practitioner or team will require a more
sophisticated approach than has hitherto been the case.

Total quality management and continuous quality improvement

In addition to external inspection, national quality awards, and
professionally orientated methods of ensuring high standards of
care (clinical audit and clinical guidelines), more general theories
concerning internal quality management and quality improvement
processes were developed and promoted throughout the 1980s and
1990s. These are generally referred to under the umbrella of total
quality management (TQM) or continuous quality improvement
(CQI) schemes. Although they have a slightly different emphasis,
the common belief is that quality improvement is an on-going
process and requires the full participation of all those working
within the organisation. TQM is:

> a way to manage the many processes which ensure these
> quality issues pervade and infiltrate every aspect of an
> organisation to improve its effectiveness . . . it involves
> whole [organisations] becoming quality sensitive and
> organised, in every department, every activity, every level
> and involves every individual . . . Ever since the NHS was
> set up, and even before this, people working in hospitals and
> in the community have been striving in different ways to
> provide good care and service; to do their best; and to look
> for improvement. TQM ensures that these efforts are
> harnessed, co-ordinated and apply to all aspects of the

*complex and diverse services which make up the NHS.
Quality will continue to increase as it is both managed and
total.* (Koch 1992)

Key aspects of TQM in healthcare include:

- standard setting and monitoring

- resource management; cost quantity and quality

- the physical environment

- risk management

- communication

- clinical audit

- training

- patient/customer focus: feedback/information

- promoting excellence in clinical care

- developing effective and efficient policies and procedures.

The TQM and CQI approaches have parallels with the more recent
initiatives to monitor and improve the performance of the NHS.
However, whilst TQM and CQI philosophies were used within
those organisations committed to quality improvement, clinical
governance places a *uniform* requirement on *all* NHS organisations
to comprehensively monitor and develop performance. Accountability for ensuring that appropriate clinical governance systems are
in place also gives added impetus to the need to consider all aspects
of service provision.

Summary

This chapter has illustrated that assessments of performance may
take a variety of formats and may focus on the whole organisation,
a part thereof or on an individual practitioner. One of the key

purposes of many of these programmes or initiatives is that they promote and recognise high-quality performance within the NHS or within the wider public sector. However, for those with a responsibility for developing a framework for performance management and clinical governance, it is also necessary to identify those cases where performance is at the trailing edge of acceptability. Although there are a number of systems in place which might serve this purpose, as Øvretveit (1999) concedes 'our traditional methods are not able to protect patients from the failures of the complex systems of care which is now our health service'. More rigorous approaches or different ways of reviewing performance might therefore be required.

Health authority performance review systems

Box II.1: Developing quality/performance management programmes: key issues

- Who are the providers of the service(s) (medics, nurses, receptionists, secondary/primary providers, etc.) and how does each interest group (user group/professional group/HA, etc.) define quality?

- On what points do the definitions of quality differ and how can any diversity of opinion be built into the assessment process in line with clinical governance?

- What roles should the different parties take within the process (role of professions/users/educationalists/HAs, etc.)?

- How can national standards (i.e. key performance indicators) be monitored and local standards developed?

- Which standards should be set (e.g. in terms of focus, local orientation, measurement – minimum, optimum, etc.) and what format will the assessment process take (internal, external)?

- There is a need to develop a dual strategy, i.e. policies and procedures are required which focus on improving the quality of the overall general practice provision and which are separate from those designed to address poor practitioner performance.

- What are the perceived benefits for those involved in the schemes, i.e. how do you get staff to participate in quality development schemes and with GPs who are deemed to be poor performers; what are the protocols for addressing their identified problems (e.g. confidentiality)?

- How will the information obtained via quality assessments be used and what processes will be triggered when monitoring indicates that standards have been failed/met/surpassed?

- How will new initiatives link with existing programmes of CPD, clinical audit, etc.?

- If a service is deemed to be substandard, what redress is there for the users of such a service?

Introduction

Section I has highlighted the issues which need to be considered by those developing any performance management programme. GP practices are the focal point for a range of services encompassing a large number of specialties (e.g. nursing, chiropody, physiotherapy, minor surgery, mental health, counselling, social work). The relationships between individual providers of care (medical or otherwise), the structures and organisations in which they work, and the quality and outcomes of patient care they provide are inter-related and are all important in the quality debate (Donabedian 1980; Gray 1992; Hutchinson 1997). Owing to the diverse nature of the services on offer, the different groups involved in the delivery of care and the complex nature of health and illness behaviour within the population it has often been suggested that quality cannot be assessed (Baker 1992). However, if quality is approached in a systematic manner, with consideration given to the range of issues outlined, then assessing performance and improving the quality of NHS care *is* possible.

Having identified the main concerns for those wishing to develop performance/quality review systems (summarised in Box II.1), Section II moves on to consider how HAs have responded to the new quality agenda. The main concern of the project upon which this book is based was to explore the range of approaches used by HAs to promote quality and to manage performance within general practice. HA initiatives developed to address poor GP performance are discussed in Chapter 4; the strategies used to monitor and develop quality within general practice are described in Chapter 5.

Chapter 4

Focusing on GP performance

With increasing emphasis being placed on improving the performance of the NHS care, all HAs have had to respond to the new
agenda and develop their policies and procedures accordingly. This
chapter, together with Chapter 5, presents the results of a national
survey of HAs[1] which looked at the strategies and schemes that they
have introduced to:

- identify and support GPs whose performance gives cause for
  concern

- monitor and develop quality in general practice and primary
  care.

Although these chapters present a particular (HA) view on how to
assess and develop performance in general practice (which may or
may not concur with views expressed by other organisations or
their representatives), the results from this survey will nonetheless
be of interest to *all* those within general practice or who are
involved in developing performance management procedures.
The issues surrounding the whole question of how to assesses
performance are of concern throughout the health sector, and this
is particularly so following the introduction of clinical governance
and revalidation.

[1] 92% of all HAs in England and Wales responded to the survey, completed in 1998. The
project was funded by the GP Unit, NHSE West Midlands and carried out by the Centre
for Health Planning and Management, Keele University.

Developing working groups to focus on performance

Almost all HAs reported that they were acutely aware of the need to address the question of GP performance following implementation of the 1995 Medical (Professional Performance) Act and recent White Papers; 76 HAs specifically mentioned that they had established a local working group to consider aspects of GP performance together with the quality of primary care services. Composition of the working groups followed a relatively common pattern – a core membership of HA representatives (typically from departments concerned with quality, commissioning, localities, and public health) together with representatives of the LMC, pharmaceutical advisors and RCGP representatives. This collaborative and multidisciplinary basis to the working groups was felt to be essential given the range of issues connected with developing quality in primary care. However, very few HAs specifically cited representatives from the professions allied to medicine as being involved in performance working groups and *no* HA mentioned lay representation (either directly or indirectly through the CHC).

This may reflect:

- the view expressed that self-regulation is the most appropriate means to ensure standards of professional practice, and the corresponding claim that non-professionals are not in a position to assess medical practice and/or

- the overriding concern of HAs, at the time, of ensuring a baseline standard of GP performance, which therefore skewed working group composition towards the inclusion of representatives from those parties directly associated with general medical practice and also

- the general concern that, for the new performance procedures to succeed, a high level of confidentiality would be required both in terms of data collection and in relation to those GPs who are identified as being 'poor performers' and who undertake remedial action.

Key questions

The working groups were addressing a wide range of questions concerning performance management:

- How do you define GP underperformance? Is it, for example, determined by what a GP does, irrespective of outcome? Is it an outcome measure, irrespective of how such outcomes are achieved? Or should what an individual practitioner does and the outcomes that are achieved both form a focus for assessment – in which case how are the two related?

- How are standards and indicators set and enforced?

- The weighting of any standards/indicators used.

- What methods are used to identify a GP who may be underperforming?

- What principles should apply to working with GPs whose performance gives cause for concern?

- How do you understand why a GP is underperforming?

- What is an appropriate outcome measure? (Health gain, mortality and/or morbidity rates, appropriate treatment, etc. could all be seen as salient outcomes, along with a number of other aspects of service provision such as equity.)

- What local interventions are required to support GPs whose performance is deemed to be poor?

- How do you resource these arrangements?

- How do you evaluate the impact of any action taken and what are the mechanisms for reporting and follow up?

Developing models of assessment for GP performance

In developing a strategy to address cases of poor individual performance, many HAs clearly recognised that the focus of debate needed to encompass a broader perspective than simply the performance of an individual practitioner. North Trent Region, for example, identified the following as being potential areas where costs might be incurred as a result of implementing the new legislation concerning poorly performing GPs.

- Infrastructure (appropriate management, systems, secretarial support, staff time).

- Superstructure (buildings, capital replacement, upgrading, equipment).

- Education (supporting GPs who are identified to be poor performers through assessment, mentoring, ongoing CME, re-certification).

- Quality assurance (promoting audit, ensuring appropriate risk management, developing mechanisms to meet the new quality agenda, i.e. to measure health outcomes, meet national performance indicators, identify health needs, etc.).

Despite widespread awareness of the need to address cases of poor professional performance amongst GPs, only a minority of HAs reported that they had introduced formal procedures with agreed criteria to identify particular GPs whose performance gave cause for concern. Where strategies and procedures had been developed and implemented (or were in the process of being established), some diversity was apparent which may reflect local custom and practice.

Examples were provided of how identification of poorly performing GPs was undertaken from basic feedback throughout the HA regarding:

- the number of complaints received about a particular doctor
- the level of target achievements
- the generic prescribing rate.

Some HAs stated that they reviewed such information on a regular basis without having developed this into more formal structures with clear standards. Indeed, a few HAs said that they still relied, in part, on *ad hoc* or 'gut' feelings about competencies. The majority of HAs, however, recognised the need to move forward on this topic although at the time of the survey many had yet to develop more formal systems of assessment. North and Mid-Hampshire HA, for example, stated that they:

> . . . *have always been aware of some GPs who provide a poorer service than others. This knowledge comes through the complaints department, and through contact with the premises by the locality managers and the pharmaceutical and medical advisors. With the advent of the new performance procedures from the GMC we have begun to think how we could work with the LMC to develop some form of peer review.*

Similarly, the approach of Dudley HA had, until recently:

> . . . *been relatively ad-hoc and informal . . . our LMC has been happy to function in a 'pastoral' role and we have invariably used the Secretary of the LMC as the first port of call if issues of poor performance have been raised with us in the past.*

Dudley, like others, typically used such information as complaints and comparative activity indicators as part of its annual practice development cycle. Along with other HAs in the West Midlands, they have been working with the Regional LMC to develop a more formalised and uniform framework for the detection and management of poorly performing GPs. Birmingham HA specifically emphasised the importance of working within a regional context. They were:

> . . . *trying to develop an effective performance monitoring system of GPs as providers that will address quality in general practice and assist in the early identification of poorly performing GPs.*

Amongst those HAs who had implemented new approaches to support GP performance, three key requirements were commonly identified during the consultation and developmental stages of this work. These centred on the need for working groups to:

- define a local process for handling the issue
- develop a diagnostic tool (with clearly defined standards and/or indicators) to assess performance
- develop an understanding of possible support networks.

Where strategies have been devised and introduced, they tend to have four distinct phases. These focus on:

- aspects of initial screening of GP performance (i.e. the collection and analysis of data which signifies that a particular GP might be giving cause for concern)
- an assessment of performance
- the development and implementation of a remedial action plan
- reassessment, with possible referral to the GMC if deemed necessary.

A number of the pilot sites – where new systems have been developed to address poor GP performance – provided information about the schemes and their experiences.

The introduction of new performance monitoring procedures

Sheffield HA

The philosophy adopted by the University of Sheffield regional working group (comprised of representatives from the local medical committees, medical audit advisory groups, CME tutors and HAs) is typical of the approach adopted by many HAs regarding the assessment of GP performance. The Sheffield working group explicitly stated that:

> The aim [of their new procedures] is . . . not to punish the doctors . . . but to determine whether performance is seriously deficient, through peer assessment, and if so, try to improve that performance using a mutually agreed development plan that incorporates adult learning techniques, retraining and counselling where appropriate.

The presumptions which the working party agreed upon were that it was the responsibility of HAs, the medical profession and allied professionals working within the primary and secondary care sectors of the NHS to identify doctors who are underperforming. In developing their strategy, the working group felt that:

> **under-performance is the repeated failure to meet acceptable standards over a period of time.**

Details were not given, however, as to what constituted an appropriate 'period of time' for assessment.

Within Sheffield, it was felt that the outcome of any procedures could be judged in terms of patient care, since the quality of service provision should improve as a result of a GP – whose performance was previously at the 'trailing edge' of acceptability – being given assistance/remedial action. However, whilst it was apparent that many HAs assumed that improved patient care would be realised, very little detail was provided as to how this might be assessed.

The Sheffield working party agreed a schedule to pilot 'proactive' support for poorly performing GPs based upon the principles that:

- doctors should be able to determine their own learning needs with the help of a mentor

- learning agendas need to include personal and public needs

- retraining should remain within an educational setting and offer opportunities for growth, support and development in areas of lesser competence

- doctors should demonstrate the ability to carry out reflective learning and to organise their time to enable this to happen

- adult learning methods are essential to foster good motivation; positive attributes should be recognised

- a programme of action should be mutually agreed with evaluation procedures with an in-built timescale

- the consequences of inertia/resistance to change/refusal to participate should be made explicit.

The following schema was derived from the working group's discussions (*see* Figure 4.1):

- Doctors giving cause for concern should be formally identified at HA level.

- Performance indicators would be used to clarify the reason for intervention.

- Each HA would liaise with a 'wise group of four' (the Performance Review Quartet consists of a medical advisor to the HA, a LMC representative, a MAAG representative and a GP tutor (CME) – all of whom will be engaged in active general practice), who would consider the information available and recommend appropriate action.

- The HA would write to the GP concerned offering a 'mentoring' visit by an approved GP tutor to discuss the area of concern and to appraise the needs of the GP. Information elicited at the visit would remain confidential to the GP and the PRQ. If progress depended on HA involvement, then agreed plans could be passed on by the GP. The GP could have a colleague sitting in on the visit.

- Failure of the GP to respond would be followed up by personal contact and a second letter.

- The visit should result in an assessment of problems and areas of need. A plan for progress within a reasonable timescale will be drawn up by the mentor and agreed with the GP. An educational assessment would be conducted if indicated (involving a second half-day visit).

- Failure to progress satisfactorily will be determined using the performance criteria at the end of the agreed timescale. Confidentiality will be maintained, but the GP will be advised that failure to achieve agreed standards may result in referral to the GMC.

Clearly defined duties for each of the main parties involved were outlined so that responsibility for key areas of action and accountability was explicit. Some funding for the Sheffield pilot project came from the Postgraduate Dean's budget, but the HA and LMC reported that they were working on identifying long-term support for the scheme.

The question of the additional funding required to develop and implement appropriate structures and mechanisms was felt to be a significant one by a number of HAs. The key stages of the new procedures (those of development, implementation and action) were regarded as placing significant demands on available resources, and the long-term support for the new procedures was seen to be a key issue. As the GP Performance Project Steering Group for South-East Thames noted, the development and implementation of the new policies and procedures:

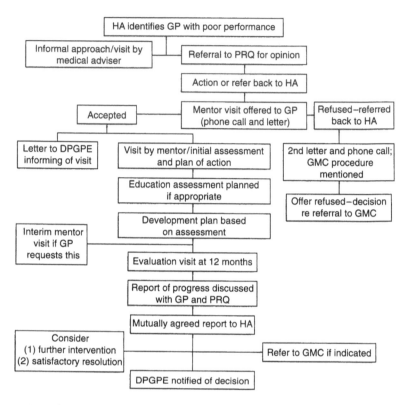

Figure 4.1 Support process for poorly performing GPs (University of Sheffield).

. . . is time consuming, energy consuming and labour intensive . . . each participant requires prolonged attention, probably over many months . . . the facilitators need the skills to work at any number of levels from knowledge, resourcing through to dealing with emotional blocking. The facilitators themselves . . . need considerable support and training.

Morecambe Bay HA

The approach adopted within Sheffield closely parallels that implemented by the North West regional office which, in 1996, sought a number of volunteer local HAs to pilot a project aimed at informing the development of health service guidance on the implementation of the 1997 Act both nationally and locally. Morecambe Bay HA (MBHA), with the agreement of the LMC, undertook one of the pilot projects. The Morecambe Bay project group had input from the LMC, the Department of Public Health (MBHA), the Director of Primary Care (MBHA), a medical advisor (MBHA), a pharmacy advisor (MBHA), a local postgraduate tutor and the Contractor Services Section (MBHA).

Two major concerns of the MBHA project group were that any outcome needed to have broad professional credibility and that matters should be dealt with in an arbitrary and even-handed way. Confidentiality had to be maintained throughout the process in order that doctors would have confidence in the new procedures. The project group:

> *worked on the premise that the performance of a doctor was not simply a clinical issue. General Practitioners are employers and have attendant legal responsibilities in this respect; in addition they are responsible for the effective working of small organisations within the health system. In its broadest sense, the environment in which a doctor works could and does have an impact on performance . . . [furthermore] although the health system has the responsibility to create an appropriate environment for successful working, doctors have their part to play in this respect.*

The MBHA project therefore focused on a broad spectrum of issues when determining whether performance gives cause for concern, taking a complementary approach to issues such as:

- the explicit requirements for HAs to develop primary care capability

- the new complaints and disciplinary procedures

- the development of a summative assessment process in the training of GP registrars

- the possible introduction of a re-validation process for NHS clinicians.

A clearly defined procedure was developed and implemented in Morecambe Bay (*see* Figure 4.2). This highlighted several sources of information which could be used to identify a GP whose performance might be regarded as falling below an acceptable standard. These sources ranged from 'soft' 'triggers' (e.g. information obtained by the HA from informal discussion with colleagues, trust staff, etc.) to 'hard' data (health targets, staff turnover, PGEA allowances, etc.). Other triggers which initiated the process included self-referral by an individual GP and complaints. Complaints were not 'automatically seen as a cause for concern' since it was felt that they might be a combination of both fact and anecdote. Isolated complaints were not necessarily felt to be a problem, and even with a number of complaints about a particular GP it was argued that a balanced view would need to be taken in the light of both the patients' and the clinicians' comments.

Once it is established that the information provided to the HA (from whatever source) gives cause for concern, GPs would be subject to assessment according to a range of HA performance indicators. It was also proposed that advice may be sought at this stage from the local GP tutor and/or, anonymously, from the LMC Chair or Secretary. The GP in question would be contacted by an appropriate facilitator, with a view to discussing whether the concern is justified and, if so, what action needs to be taken. A structured discussion tool was developed by MBHA in order to both aid this part of the process and also to ensure that consistency and professional acceptance were maintained. The outcome of such a meeting provides the basis for a report for both the doctor and the HA, and is shared with those who are involved in supporting, developing and implementing the action plan to improve the GP's performance. Once this has been completed (within the agreed timescale) meetings are held to determine whether the action plan has been met, and a confidential report is submitted to the HA.

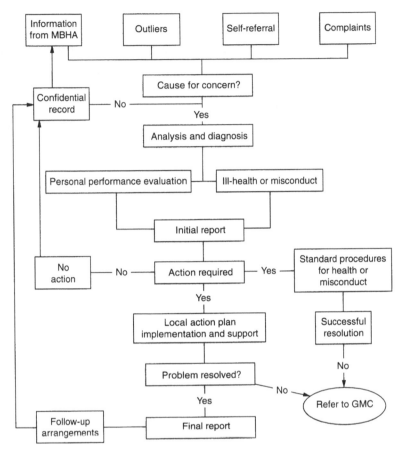

Figure 4.2   Process flow chart for poorly performing GPs (Morecambe Bay, HA).

Arrangements are made for on-going practical and educational professional support for the GP.

A number of key sources of support for individual practitioners were identified, dependent upon whether those at the centre of the process wished to use them. These included, for example, local GP tutors, the HA's primary care development team, the RCGP local faculty and directors of postgraduate practice education.

What we see therefore in both Morecambe Bay and Sheffield, is the need to develop clearly defined procedures for addressing aspects of professional performance. The two cases also emphasise that any review programme needs to have, built into it, specific criteria (against which performance is assessed) and some threshold which triggers further review and assessment. Whilst the data gathered may take the form of soft data (such as informal discussions or gut feelings which may be valuable sources of information, taken in conjunction with more substantive data) most HAs were looking to introduce clear standards and indicators against which performance could be assessed.

Indicators to assess GP performance

As we have seen, the use of indicators to assess the relative quality of health service provision has received much attention following publication of the consultation document *The New NHS: Modern Dependable. A National Framework for Assessing Performance* (DoH 1998b), and debate continues as to their appropriateness, relevance and focus (Campbell *et al.* 1997; Roland 1997; Davies and Lampel 1998; Grenville 1998; Sheldon 1998).

In developing ways to assess the quality of GP-based or primary care a number of HAs sought to define what is meant by 'poor performance' or 'poor quality' and, more significantly, how this might be detected. The use of standards and indicators to determine which GPs are deemed to be at the 'trailing edge of acceptable performance' constituted a principal focus of attention for many HAs in the development of a local strategy (SE Thames, North Staffordshire), although in line with the wider debate regarding the use of indicators at a national level, concern was expressed by several respondents as to the validity of indicators to directly assess competency, together with the problems inherent in collating the relevant information in a meaningful way. The South-East Thames Region GP Performance Project Steering Group, for example, felt that:

> standards should only be set within areas of activity for which accurate data was available . . . and that the

performance standards set would, at best, provide a fairly
superficial indication of more general under performance.
Failure to meet the standards set would do no more than
trigger the need for further enquiry.

Despite such concerns, a number of HAs reported that they were either in the process of developing or using a range of indicators against which to assess performance.

North Derbyshire Health (amongst others) provided details of the performance criteria and minimum standards that they were considering using. A key factor as to which criteria might be selected to assess performance from a HA perspective appears to be access to information about GP activity, since, for all of the criteria proposed by North Derbyshire Health, a defined individual within the HA was able to provide information relative to that standard.

The proposed performance indicators shown in Table 4.1 cover both a doctor's performance and associated factors (premises, WTE staff, etc.). However, no information was provided as to how the indicators relate to each other and what triggers are required. That is to say, would failure in one assessment category lead to a doctor being classed as 'poorly performing' or do several factors need to occur simultaneously before any action is taken? Also, are the indicators given equal weight or are those related directly to professional competencies (such as the PGEA) given greater consideration than, for example, substandard premises? It is worthy of note that after considerable discussion by the HA and LMCs in both North and South Derbyshire 'these indicators were roundly criticised at a meeting of interested parties' and were *not* implemented (Grenville 1998).

The issue of the comparative importance of different indicators was highlighted by South-East Thames, who provided details of the indicators that they were currently using and the relative scoring for each one (*see* Table 4.2). However, even where consideration

Table 4.1   Proposed performance indicators (North Derbyshire) (derived from the work undertaken by ScHARR)

Performance criteria	Proposed minimal standard
Complaints	Doctors who have had two or more formal complaints upheld against them by a service committee
Cervical cytology (targets)	GPs achieving less than 30% of the target group
Immunisations	GPs achieving less than 40% of the target group for immunisation of under two-year-olds and 20% of the target group for under five-year-olds
Patients leaving the practice	GPs registering more than a 2.5% deviation from the HA average for patients leaving the practice without changing address
Return of medical records	GPs returning fewer than 50% of medical records within three months of first request
Staffing levels	GPs who have fewer than one WTE member of staff per 1000 patients
Premises	GPs where remission of rent/rates have been agreed due to poor standard of premises
PGEA	GPs who have made no PGEA claim within the previous two years
Comparative referral rates	Information to be gathered on those GPs who are referring very small numbers of patients
Availability of doctor	Information is held that highlights those GPs who are constantly being deputised for due to health problems and whose patient contact time is low
Clinical effectiveness/audit	Issues around clinical effectiveness can be checked with Mr X
Health promotion	Information is held which would identify those practices who do not hold CDM clinics
Prescribing doctors in the top 5% for:	• antidiarrhoeals • appetite suppressants • barbiturates
Doctors in the bottom 5% for:	• cardiovascular drugs • asthma drugs • antidiabetics
Doctors where . . .	. . . the DDD ratio of inhaled steroids to bronchodilators is below 0.33 (ACTAP)

Table 4.1   *(cont.)*

Performance criteria	Proposed minimal standard
	. . . DDDs of hypnotics and anxiolytics per 1000 adjusted prescribe units exceed 6910 (ACTAP) . . . the top 5 NSAIDS issued account for less than 85% of the NSAIDS prescribed (ACTAP)

Key:
DDD (defined daily dose)   ACTAP (Audit Committee-Treatment and Prescribing)
NSAIDS (non-steroidal anti-inflammatory drugs)   PGEA (postgraduate education allowance)

has been given to this, it was unclear whether a threshold needed to be broken to instigate action.

Limitations of standards and indicators

Some degree of caution needs to be exercised when using indicators as a gauge of professional performance. The apparently common use of the PGEA claim as a potential indicator of 'poor' performance (*see* Tables 4.1 and 4.2) highlights the point in question. The PGEA varies throughout the country and has generally not been monitored or standardised. There is wide variation regarding the nature of the courses which qualify for PGEA, a situation which led to a review of the PGEA by the Chief Medical Officer (Working Party on Continuous Professional Development). It is likely that the PGEA will change in the future to become more of a practice-based, multiprofessional, learning-based system, with personal and professional development plans. Consequently, whilst a low level of PGEA claims may identify those individuals who lack recent professional development, claiming full PGEA allowance does not automatically infer uniformity of standards or competencies.

Whilst performance indicators may be used to identify those practitioners whose practice deviates from a given norm or standard (Majeed and Voss 1995), such indicators only measure

Table 4.2   Performance indicators with weightings (South-East Thames)

Indicator	Criteria	Weighting
Complaints	GPs who, during the last three years, have had two or more formal complaints against them upheld by a medical services committee and not overturned on appeal	Two confirmed complaints scores 1 point, each additional complaint scores an extra point
Cervical cytology	GPs/practices achieving less than 30% of target group (to include cervical cytology from all sources)	1 point
Immunisation (1)	GPs/practices achieving less than 40% of target group for immunisation of under two-year-olds (from all sources)	1 point
Immunisation (2)	GPs/practices achieving less than 20% of target group for immunisation of under five-year-olds (from all sources)	1 point
Patients leaving practice	GPs/practices registering more than 2.5% above the FHSA average for patients leaving the practice without changing address	1 point
Premises	GPs/practices where any remission of rents and rates remuneration has been agreed by LMC and FHSA	1 point
Return of notes	GPs/practices returning fewer than 50% of medical record envelopes within three months of first request	1 point
Staff	GPs/practices with a list of more than 1000 patients who have less than one member of reimbursable employed staff for the main practice	1 point
PGEA	GPs who have made no PGEA allowance within the previous two years	2 points
Prescribing	Practices in the top 5% for the prescribing of antidiarrhoeals	1/2 point
	Practices in the top 5% for the prescribing of appetite suppressants	1/2 point
	Practices in the top 5% for the prescribing of barbiturates	1/2 point

Table 4.2 (*cont.*)

Indicator	Criteria	Weighting
	Practices where the DDD ratio of inhaled steroids to bronchodilators is below 0.33 (ACTAP)	1/2 point
	Practices where the top five NSAIDS used in the practice account for less than 85% of the NSAIDS prescribed	1/2 point
	Practices where DDDs of hypnotics and anxiolytics per 1000 adjusted prescribing units exceeds 6910 (ACTAP)	1/2 point
	Practices in the bottom 5% for the prescribing of cardiovascular/asthma/ antidiabetic drugs	1/2 point each

Key:
DDD (defined daily dose)   ACTAP (Audit Committee-Treatment and Prescribing)
NSAIDS (non-steroidal anti-inflammatory drugs)   PGEA (postgraduate education allowance)

certain aspects of performance and may not, for example, provide an assessment of the clinical care of patients, nor do they relate to the appropriateness of such care (Campbell *et al.* 1997). Equally, the characteristics of both the population and of the configuration of services in any locality may have an impact on the ability to meet specific local or national targets (Giuffrida *et al.* 1999). It might also be the case that, through introducing certain indicators, HAs, PCGs and practitioners concentrate on improving only those indicators about which data are being collected rather than improving the overall quality of their care. The widespread and sometimes heated debates surrounding indicators show no sign of abating and one can only envisage that, with changing service configurations and more detailed analysis, this situation will continue into the foreseeable future.

The purpose of indicators is also significant. There are two distinct approaches which could be applied when determining a focus for assessment, each of which impacts on the quality process.

The first approach uses indicators which are concerned with assessing what GPs are actually doing, irrespective of the outcome. The second approach focuses on the outcomes of care, and is not primarily concerned with how such outcomes are achieved. In examining the performance of GPs, either or both approaches might apply, and it is important that discussions on professional performance include consideration of this matter.

It is also important to develop indicators which have a specific purpose, as opposed to merely developing indicators from current data sets (such as Exeter or PACT). Whilst the information contained in such data sets *may* give a good indication about the nature of services provided and of individual practices, it is typically practice orientated, and untangling the contribution of the individual to such returns may be difficult. Equally, and particularly so in the case of single-handed GPs, certain services may be provided by neighbouring practices (e.g. child health surveillance). Hence an indicator data set may highlight that certain core services are not being provided whilst, in practice, arrangements have been made for provision elsewhere. In this context, the indicator data set can only be used as a guide and further enquiry is necessary to uncover the root causes for apparent poor performance.

The data sets must be appropriate for assessments of perform-ance and should be collected and presented in a format which facilitates ease of analysis. If this is not the case, as recent research in some HAs suggests (Birch and Scrivens 1999), then new data sets and revised ways of data collection and analysis must be considered.

The importance of clinical involvement, credibility and influence

With a move away from examining the context within which care is delivered, to one which directly assesses the provision and appropriateness of care and includes some form of outcome assessment, greater involvement of professional groups is required. Whilst 76 HAs acknowledged the need to collaborate with the professions in local working groups, it is a matter of concern that the remainder of respondents did not specifically cite the existence of such multidisciplinary groups. Close collaboration and partnership between the HA, local GPs, PCGs, LMCs, the RCGP and GP tutors is essential to address the issues of poor GP performance and the quality of care provided, as highlighted by Morecambe Bay HA. Additionally, as Lincolnshire HA recognised, obtaining the support of local practitioners is essential if one is to effect changes in professional attitudes and behaviour, since, '[peer] influence is a key determinant of general practitioner . . . change'.

Crucial to the success of any quality programme is the willingness of clinicians (and, of course, the professions allied to medicine and other NHS staff) to be involved. Historically, most quality assurance programmes have found this difficult to achieve. All of the organisational accreditation systems (in both the UK and elsewhere), for example, have faced the same problem of obtaining the willing participation of doctors. The solution has tended to focus on the production of information which is of relevance to clinicians – that is, more clinically related information – and to recast the basic approach to meet demands for greater flexibility in the management of quality. The result has been an acceptance that quality is better communicated through education and persuasion rather than central dicta. Similarly, within the UK, the new procedures developed to address cases of poor GP performance are based on the premise that re-education and training will, in the majority of cases, remedy the situation. The importance of continuing professional development in combating poor performance was highlighted by some HAs and should gain higher prominence following the Chief Medical Officer's review of CPD and the White Paper, *A First Class Service* (DoH 1998a).

Causes of poor performance

Although much of the literature supplied in response to the survey reflected a keen awareness of the need to develop local indicators to determine in which area (if any) GPs are felt to be underperforming, few HAs explicitly underpinned this with potential reasons as to *why* GPs did not perform well. A useful adjunct to this is the documentation provided by South-East Thames and South Cheshire. South-East Thames hypothesised that there are five reasons as to why under-performance may occur.

1 **Ignorance**

   At one end of the spectrum, people will fail to perform simply because they do not know something or they have forgotten it. Changes in medical practices and the role of GPs may lead, over a period of time, to a cumulative failure to acquire essential new knowledge.

2 **Knowing but not understanding**

   It is possible to memorise facts without truly understanding their meaning. It is necessary to examine the context and logic of knowledge – to relate it to that which is previously known or which is being experienced. It is necessary to think through its implications. To be useful in a variety of situations knowledge needs to be restructured and reshaped in a way which is personally usable.

3 **Having competence but failing in performance**

   Performance involves using competencies in a variety of situations to take account of context. It requires the demonstration of a competence, or more often a sequence of competencies, in an appropriate way which demands sequencing and judgement . . . The standards of performance expected may well vary from place to place and time to time; GPs who daily have to perform in poorly equipped buildings with low levels of staffing are bound to find it harder to maintain high levels of care. Central to turning competence into performance is the ability to learn from experience. The transformation of experience by reflection, the formation of concepts and the testing of the implications of those concepts in new situations is at the heart of developing the skills of the practitioner.

4 **Lacking motivation**

The doctor who is perfectly able to perform well, may not do so simply because motivation is lost. In some cases it may never have been present to begin with. Lack of motivation may derive from external sources (e.g. an excessive workload or inadequate financial reward) or internal sources (e.g. poor self image or an inability to seek or gain reward).

5 **Being prevented from performing**

Some doctors have the competence, can perform, wish to perform, but then get blocked. Again, these blocks may be external (e.g. lack of resources – poor building, inadequate staff, insufficient information) or internal (e.g. lack of confidence, perceived lack of expertise).

South Cheshire Health listed possible reasons for underperformance as being those of:

- isolation
- poor preparation for general practice
- lack of involvement in meaningful continuing education
- stress
- poor organisation
- low morale
- poor infrastructure
- under-resourced
- poor support (from, for example, the HA)
- physical and/or mental illness.

Added to this, Campbell *et al.* (1997) argue that:

> *environmental factors such as socio-demographic charac-*
> *teristics of the population are known to have a major effect*
> *on, for example, cervical cytology rates. Quality indicators*
> *do not define the cause of a problem: they identify an issue*
> *which may require further investigation.*

It is essential in addressing the question of performance in general practice to bear in mind that problems may lie with the individual (through lack of training and education), with the practice (the organisation/prescribing patterns), with the HA (lack of invest-ment) or outwith the control of either GP, practice or HA (e.g. in relation to screening uptake).

High quality performance

Whilst discussion has so far focused on HA initiatives to tackle the problem of poorly performing GPs there are, as Section I has highlighted, professionally orientated national schemes which seek to recognise the *high* quality of care offered by individual practitioners. The RCGP, for example, has a number of pro-grammes which are regarded as promoting high-quality physician care and are seen as 'gold' standards within the profession (i.e. Membership and Fellowship of the RCGP).

Although HA attention appears to concentrate on those GPs at the other end of the spectrum, whose performance gives cause for concern, there is no reason why the precepts upon which the Membership and Fellowship by Assessment are based could not be incorporated into HA and PCG strategies to develop GP perform-ance. That is to say, the methodologies, targets and standards set by the RCGP in its own assessment of professional performance could be both promoted within and supported by HAs and PCGs as an integral part of their overall performance assessment programme.

Summary

Much of the documentation submitted illustrated that the large majority of HAs had, at the very least, begun discussions about the need for new policies and procedures to identify and deal with the question of poor performance amongst GPs. A smaller number had progressed this to a point of implementation. However, the problems of moving from a theoretical perspective to implementing a strategy and effecting change were highlighted as being considerable (St Helens and Knowsley HA).

From an analysis of the ways in which HAs are tackling the issue of poorly performing GPs, it is evident that a number of different approaches exist to assess and monitor GP performance (e.g. Birmingham, North Staffordshire, South Staffordshire, Sandwell, Barnet, Salford and Trafford, North and Mid-Hampshire, Cambridge and Huntingdon). Some HAs appear content to rely on existing mechanisms, others have developed in-house procedures, whilst a number are looking towards an agreed regional procedure for tackling the problem.

The need to develop and implement an approach which is rigorous and acceptable both within the HA area and to a wider audience was felt to be an important consideration, and this path has been favoured in a number of areas. Within the West Midlands, for example, the majority of HAs have now committed themselves to a regional approach (personal communication 1999) – thereby paralleling the regional perspectives of the North West and North Trent.

In general, where new procedures have been developed, HAs reported that the indicators of poor performance had been drawn up by a project team combining a range of professionals, although little information was given regarding the remit of the team and the level at which consultation occurred with practitioners in the local area (both the medical profession and those allied to medicine). Assessment of individual performance is typically that of peer review (e.g. the North Trent Performance Review Quartet consisted of individuals who were all active in general practice), and the resulting progress of any action to remedy poor performance is held by the HA and not made public.

Where more formalised structures and indicators have been developed, there is some degree of congruence between the indicators which are being used to assess GP performance. A comparison of the proposed indicators for North Derbyshire/ South-East Thames and the discussion paper for developing structures within Birmingham HA, for example, shows that the performance targets are very similar. The concerns raised regarding acceptable and appropriate indicators and the need to ensure credibility and widespread professional concurrence are also similar.

Whilst the review of HA strategies highlighted that considerable attention is being given to the question of poor performance, it remains the case that there may be those GPs who deliver care which falls short of average standards but who are not yet at the 'trailing edge of acceptability'. For those involved in developing the quality of general practice-based care, it is also important to identify these individuals and to seek to improve performance across the board. For example, if a normal distribution curve exists in the area of GP performance and competency as shown in Figure 4.3 (although no national or local data are currently available on this), then the new GMC procedures targeted at the most severe cases of poor performance are directed at only the tip of the iceberg of those GPs whose performance falls below an average standard. Furthermore, whilst much HA attention is being given to those GPs whose performance is at the 'trailing edge of acceptable performance' (B in Figure 4.3), again this neglects the potentially large number of GPs whose performance may be 'below average' (C in Figure 4.3).

Even if the distribution curve regarding GP performance is skewed (in either a positive or negative direction), the major concern for those charged with implementing clinical governance

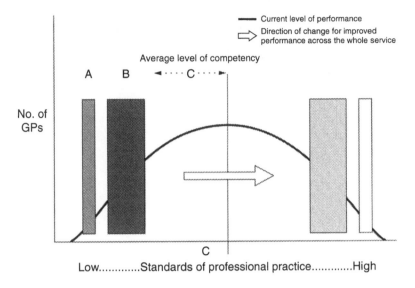

Key:

A = small number of GPs whose professional performance fails to improve following local measures and who are referred to GMC

B = relatively small number of GPs whose performance is sufficiently poor to initiate local procedure and where improvement occurs without redress to GMC

C = larger proportion of GPs whose performance falls below the local average standard but which is not sufficiently poor to initiate local procedures

D = GPs whose performance comes under scrutiny as part of a practice quality assessment and which, as part of such an assessment, is deemed to be of 'quality'

E = GPs whose individual performance is assessed and is deemed to be of high quality, i.e. RCGP Fellowship by Assessment

Figure 4.3   Normal distribution curve for GP performance.

and developing performance should be how one improves the totality of GP performance. This requires a knowledge of both the relationships between individual performance, organisational context, environment (i.e. socio-demographic factors) and the nature of service provision throughout the district, which itself encompasses a broader remit than simply focusing on a small number of under performing individuals.

Given that an individual's performance may be affected both by the organisation and the context within which he or she works, the remit of many of the HA working groups went beyond simply addressing the question of poorly performing GPs and considered the development of quality in general practice *per se.* As Rosenthal (1995) notes, widespread variation exists in respect of local regulation, and clinical governance cannot be run centrally. It has to start with every doctor, every clinical team and every PCG – which leads to the whole issue of how one assesses the performance of an organisation.

Chapter 5

Quality in general practice

Recent policy initiatives place particular emphasis on the role that primary care providers will play in delivering the new health agenda. However, for those responsible for developing and implementing effective performance management or quality review procedures, practice-based primary care poses particular difficulties due to a number of factors. The diverse nature of service provision both within and between localities, the lack of common organisational structures, changing service configurations and the range of professional and contractual relationships which occur, all complicate matters. However, all PCGs (future PCTs) and HAs are having to address issues of performance management and quality improvement in general practice, and this chapter reviews the range of current approaches and concludes by drawing together the key issues facing commissioners and providers as they develop their quality management strategies.

Reviewing quality

All HAs responding to the survey indicated that they monitored quality in general practice, although the approach, policies and procedures adopted to achieve this varied considerably. Several methods, ranging from informal practice visits and the routine collection of data to specific quality awards and comprehensive local programmes for quality development were reported. Many HAs indicated that they were in the process of developing a more rigorous approach to the monitoring of quality within general practice. For example, West Hertfordshire HA commented that:

> the HA has recognised the need to develop a more systematic approach to performance management of general practice in its provider role. As part of the work in developing a framework for performance management, a small working group has been looking at performance indicators and the process that could be used to implement a revised framework in [this] HA.[1]

HAs reported that they used a number of formal and informal approaches to monitor the quality of local service provision. As Box 5.1 illustrates, the range of techniques that were used (often in conjunction with other methods) showed a high degree of variation.

Local quality initiatives

Single methods alone are not generally used to assess service provision. The majority of HAs reported that a range of measures are used simultaneously, thereby allowing them to gain an overall picture of the performance of practices within a district. Some HAs reported that quality in general practice was monitored according to baseline data, routinely collected from various sources. These frequently included the number of complaints recorded (inclusive of those dealt with via 'in-house' mechanisms and also those made to the HA) and data obtained through the GP payment scheme which records activity such as cervical cytology (smears), childhood immunisation, child health surveillance, female contraception, maternity care provided, vaccinations and night visits.

[1] The HA quotes are unpublished written accounts which were provided in response to the research programme.

Box 5.1: Examples of some of the methodologies used by HAs for monitoring quality in general practice

- In-house benchmarking (e.g. Walsall)

- Primary care benchmarking (a total of 23 HAs including Shropshire, Morecambe Bay, Leicestershire, Sunderland and Wiltshire; for a complete list *see* Rodger and Watkins 1999), through the benchmarking 'club', took part in first round of a nationally orientated project

- Practice profiling (e.g. North Cumbria, Isle of Wight)

- Locality profiling (e.g. Lincolnshire)

- Practice visits in conjunction with other mechanisms (e.g. North Staffordshire, Camden and Islington)

- Developing a primary care clinical effectiveness programme (e.g. East Kent)

- The use of the King's Fund Organisational Audit (KFOA) programme (Camden and Islington)

- The development of local accreditation programmes (e.g. Northumberland, Sheffield and Leicestershire)

- Local quality schemes (e.g. Bedfordshire, Solihull, South Derbyshire, Portsmouth and South East Hampshire, Lambeth, Southwark and Lewisham)

- London initiative zone funding was made available for the development of primary care in the capital and was used in some cases to facilitate workforce flexibilities and to provide educational incentives for local GPs

---

A large number of HAs have developed more advanced performance review and quality development strategies, which incorporate a number of different techniques. Northumberland HA, for example, not only utilise routine data but have developed a range of tools which they feel enables them to 'quickly build up a comprehensive picture and identify particular areas of poor performance'.

These include:

- an accountability framework for those GPs who were fundholders

- developing the Northumberland practice accreditation programme

- introducing a nurse development programme

- a prescribing strategy

- the development of a self-assessment tool for primary health care teams

- a competencies framework

- clinical audit

- promoting participation in the KFOA

- the development of primary care partnership.

Meanwhile, Lambeth, Southwark and Lewisham emphasised that, *inter alia*, key priorities of their practice development programme would be:

- developing primary care services according to the needs of the local population

- developing standards and quality indicators for primary care

- encouraging all practices to participate in their local practice quality initiative and to develop their service in line with band C (the HA operates a quality banding scheme).

No two HA responses were identical, although the measures used to determine quality within primary care or general practice included some that were used more frequently than others (e.g. quality development schemes, practices visits, reviews of prescribing, primary care development groups). The following section presents examples of a number of differing techniques which have been developed to determine quality in general practice.[2]

[2] Such illustrative examples do not imply that these are the *only* methods applied within a particular HA, rather they are used to illustrate the *types* of methodologies in use.

Practice surveys (e.g. Kingston and Richmond Health)

Patient (satisfaction) surveys are often used to elicit data about perceptions of care throughout the NHS (Mason 1989; Poole and Birch 1996), although the validity and reliability of such methods has been criticised (Fitzpatrick *et al.* 1984; Poole and Birch 1997). Nonetheless, such surveys, if conducted rigorously, provide salient information for HAs and practitioners who are seeking to develop service provision (and often it is the *only* method of finding out information on sensitive issues). It was upon this premise that Kingston and Richmond Health, in 1992, developed a random questionnaire survey of patients from GP practices, focusing on issues of service quality.

> *Having analysed the data we . . . prepared reports for each individual practice whereby their performance was compared with the aggregated performance for Kingston and Richmond as a whole. We also selected a number of key issues and benchmarked practices against these. This was followed up by visits to each practice to discuss their survey results with them and also to find out how they intended to use the information provided to improve performance.*

Whilst no specific examples are given, the HA commented that their efforts to find out the views of service users, and through a sharing of information 'led to the development of a number of quality initiatives in many practices'. Following on from this, the HA:

> *are always attempting to . . . rank GPs against their local peers . . . We have been able to identify a number of areas which relate to performance, but have found it extremely difficult to give due weighting to each of these. It has also been extremely difficult to disentangle quality from quantity.*

The HA did not indicate whether they have developed a district-wide scheme for standards in general practice, although they stated that they were looking to the Health Services Accreditation primary care programme as a means to develop primary care services.

The use of questionnaire surveys to develop services represents one model for quality development. However, such methods may lack professional support since the views expressed by service users are not necessarily balanced against provider and commissioner views, and there may be difficulties in arriving at a consensus regarding which areas need to be tackled on a district-wide basis. Furthermore, it should be remembered that satisfaction does not necessarily equate to service quality. Patients not only have a tendency to report high levels of overall satisfaction (which therefore masks particular areas of concern) but equally, when considering particular elements of service provision, individuals may be highly satisfied with an aspect of service provision which is of relatively little importance to them and dissatisfied with a feature which *they* perceive of as crucial (Poole and Birch 1997). It has been noted that:

> *effectively managing service quality requires a clear understanding of what service quality means to the consumer . . . [and to achieve this one] must understand the nature of customer satisfaction, service quality and customer value, and how these factors interact.* (Rust and Oliver 1994)

It is also the case that 'improving the quality of service requires managing the service product, the service environment and the service delivery' (Rust and Oliver 1994).

As many authors have noted, to achieve improvements in the quality of service requires the commitment and support of the professionals involved and, in turn, a degree of 'ownership' over projects and local directives (Øvretveit 1993). Kingston and Richmond Health, for example, have attempted to involve professionals in the quality process through visits, support and benchmarking but, even so, they still note that difficulties have been encountered.

Practice visits/annual practice development plans

HA practice visits were frequently mentioned as a prominent means to assess the provision of general practice-based care. Such visits were typically seen as occasions for information sharing, problem solving and informal peer review, rather than to determine performance against a set of locally agreed standards. Whilst practice visits were often regarded as *informal* monitoring systems, they were viewed as playing a highly significant role, since they provided opportunities to 'unpack' aspects of performance and to discuss service provision (Sandwell HA).

North Staffordshire HA undertake practice visits as part of their review of primary care services. Visits are conducted independently by members of primary and community care development, by pharmaceutical and medical advisers and by the Associate Director of GP Services. The former are chiefly concerned with the organisation, premises and staffing of the practice, whilst the latter has a broad remit of enquiry, including issues of medical management and prescribing. They do, however, note that 'when particular concerns are felt, [discussions] may be more focused' but no uniform standards and means of assessment are provided regarding what constitutes a 'good' practice or optimal performance. The visits are informal, reported back to the practice and recorded on file at the HA. In some cases, practice visits linked into the production and feedback of a practice's annual development plan, but no specifics were given as to how this fits into the overall HA or PCG strategy for quality improvement. Since the initial survey, as part of their on-going performance review package, North Staffordshire have piloted a set of performance indicators for poorly performing GPs, and are seeking to develop a more formal approach to performance monitoring in general practice.

Quality handbooks

A number of HAs indicated that they have begun to develop more structured mechanisms for assessing the quality of GP-based services. Croydon Health had recently established a primary care quality group and had produced a manual to help practices look at how they might:

> develop and apply the principles of quality assurance to general practice. It provides an overview of quality assurance in general, and offers suggestions regarding the process of implementing quality assurance tools and techniques. While the principles . . . apply to all aspects of general practice, the actual application of the theory will be influenced directly by the environment and nature of practice workloads.

The Croydon Health manual offers sample templates for quality standards under the following headings:

* organisation

* interface

* clinical practice

* environment.

Under this scheme, each practice completes those quality schedules which are deemed appropriate to it, thereby allowing for considerable local variation. Although templates are given, such standards are not regarded as definitive and 'each practice will apply some, all or, indeed, add to the list of topics provided'. A standards' format is provided to assist practices in developing standards and covers:

* critical structure

* management requirements

* standards criteria

- audit process

- audit data

- responsible person.

(Although 'audit data' is given as a category, the documentation does not detail the scope and nature of the audit.)

Moving away from a model in which practices set their own standards and assess compliance, one finds examples of schemes whereby HAs have, in conjunction with LMCs and other agencies, set broad common standards for general practice. The assessment may be informal or undertaken from outside the practice.

Health authority quality schemes

Healthy Practices Scheme (Portsmouth and South East Hampshire)

Portsmouth and South East Hampshire HA have, like many HAs, developed an approach which favours voluntary participation in quality development rather than 'the big stick' approach. Their Healthy Practices Scheme offers support to those primary care practices wishing to structure their reviews of the policies and procedures specifically designed to ensure that the practice runs smoothly. The scheme was developed over an 18-month period and involved seven primary care practices throughout the HA and the public health, quality and development directorates of the HA. It covers what are regarded as four of the most critical areas for successful general practice (health and safety of the environment, access for patients to primary health services, communication with patients and primary care teamwork) and practices enter the scheme at either of two levels:

Level 1 Practices use the scheme to assess themselves against the criteria, with support and advice from the HA as required. On submission of the completed pro-forma, practices receive a certificate of participation.

Level 2 Practices complete level 1 and the evidence they submit is validated by a colleague from another practice and/or members of the HA, as agreed with the practice. This entitles the participating practice to a certificate of achievement (if the evidence is validated) and a grant of £100 to be spent within the practice on materials, equipment or information which encourages more healthy life-styles for their practice population.

This model, whereby standards are set locally, and adherence to such standards is self-administered within practices (although there is an opportunity for external validation by a local peer group) represents one model for quality improvement. Practices who participate at level 2 of the scheme may be regarded as undertaking a local form of accreditation.

More recently, in an attempt to involve all practices in the process of quality development, Portsmouth and South East Hampshire HA have added specific indicators to their healthy practices programme. The comparative indicators they use in their SIMPLE (shared information for measurement of primary care for local evaluation) strategy cover:

- patient data (12 indicators)
- staffing (5 indicators)
- cytology (3 indicators)
- immunisations (2 indicators)
- activity (4 indicators)
- hospital procedures (2 indicators)
- prescribing (9 indicators)
- referrals for hospital admission (1 indicator)
- finance (11 indicators).

These were circulated to all GPs on the premise that such information would encourage a large number of practices to review their current policies and procedures, leading to improvements in quality. This assumption is being reviewed, since the opinion is that 'good' practices will naturally want to improve, whilst 'trailing' practices will need further impetus for change.

Wolverhampton HA provides a further example of how the process of quality development moves from an informal to a more formal strategy. Under the West Midlands region's Q1 themed review, the performance management of GPs and primary care was a major area highlighted for development by the HA which received funding from the NHS Executive. As a baseline, the HA were asked to complete a self-audit questionnaire to ascertain current activity for GP-based services, and the HA were 'currently considering [more formal] systems from elsewhere and seeing how [they] could use the base part of these to develop [their] own approach'. At the time of the study, Wolverhampton HA used a range of data to assess the performance of primary care. Although validation was not yet in place for all of the target areas, they were clearly looking to develop a more comprehensive and formally assessed programme. This is evidenced by their participation in a pilot project (along with North Staffordshire HA) funded by the NHS Executive (West Midlands) which is seeking to develop an indicator set against which general practice performance can be assessed.

Once one moves away from the more informal methods of monitoring service quality (e.g. reviewing complaints, ad hoc surveys, self-administered quality reviews) more formalised structures and processes inevitably emerge – although variation is apparent between HAs. As the SIMPLE strategy in Portsmouth and South East Hampshire illustrates, as certain initiatives develop they often expand outwith their original aims and boundaries.

Practice development planning (Northamptonshire HA)

Northamptonshire HA have developed a number of initiatives with the aim of improving the quality of general practice. For several years they, as with many other HAs, have operated a process of practice development planning (PDP) whereby each practice has a formal meeting with HA staff to discuss the short- and medium-term needs of the practice. The practice then produces a plan which ideally should include:

- the needs of the practice

- strategic direction of the practice

- resources required to take the practice forward.

This process has enabled practices to 'take a more rounded, less *ad hoc* view of their development'.

To complement the PDPs, the HA have developed a self-assessment tool, *'Recognising organisational quality in general practice'*, and they have been working with the Public Health Resource Unit in Oxford to develop a similar tool *'Recognising clinical quality'*. *'Recognising organisational quality in general practice'* was developed by the HA in conjunction with the local LMC and contains a series of organisational quality indicators for use in general practices in the area. That is to say, the indicators refer to the organisational issues that underpin the delivery of clinical services. They do not include aspects of clinical quality. The HA note that:

> *whilst the quality of clinical care is paramount, this is currently being addressed by the profession through the development of re-accreditation . . . It was acknowledged that effective clinical care is easier to provide if the organisational and management infrastructure is functioning well,*

(thereby paralleling the founding principles of accreditation systems within the hospital sector).

Practices are encouraged to make extensive use of the *'Recognising organisational quality in general practice'* pack on the basis that it focuses on the quality of management, staff and organisational systems and seeks to ensure that they are right for the services that are provided. The aim of the indicators 'is to help practices identify where they are now, what they have already achieved and where it would be useful to improve on any aspect of the practice's organisation'. The indicators have been set at two levels – **minimum** and **desirable.**

- **Minimum level** indicators are something that every practice is expected to achieve. The practice may already have reached the minimum levels, or it may need to take action, invest or develop an area to achieve them. In the initial stages it is unlikely any practice will achieve all minimum level indicators.

- **Desirable level** indicators are set above the minimum level. The practice may have already reached that level, or decide to achieve it in one or two areas.

The indicators are divided into six main areas, with a number of different topics in each:

1 **Relationships with patients** – patient records and results, access, services, information and patient participation.
2 **Management of risks** – legislation, business continuity, corporate governance and finance, complaints, services, people, infection control, premises and systems.
3 **Physical resources** – premises and equipment.
4 **Staff** – employment, locums, training and development, complaints and suggestions, administrative procedures.
5 **Teamwork** – definition and communication.
6 **Practice development and quality management** – responding to change, practice development planning, financial and resources planning and management, audit and professional development.

The aim is to ensure that a minimum level of quality is achieved in every practice across the county. Whilst the 'Recognising organisational quality in general practice' scheme is not compulsory, all practices have been asked by the HA to complete the self-assessment and to return a summary sheet to the HA. Locality teams then review these returns as part of the PDPs. Each year, practices are asked to review the indicators, adjusting their self-evaluation as appropriate. There may be some variation year on year in the indicators based on feedback and changing circumstances. However, it is seen as a 'building' process; it is not necessary to start from scratch each time.

Benchmarking for general practice (Walsall HA)

Similarly, Walsall HA noted that in order to ensure that the provision of service is:

> appropriate [for the change towards a primary care led NHS, they] now need to have a more formal approach to assessing services in primary care . . . most practices are visited frequently by staff on specific issues. A programme of GP fundholding performance reviews was run for the past two years, which led to the development of the successful GPFH benchmarking project, with a strong educational focus. Walsall has good information systems and recent work on acuity has improved the capability to produce primary care information, but further development work is required. These existing activities and proposed developments need to be brought together into a coherent programme to help the dialogue with GPs.

They have produced a draft programme which seeks to support the development of primary care. The strategy builds on the work undertaken by Moores Rowland Consulting which, as part of the GP accountability framework, developed assessment (for GPFH) by applying best practice benchmarking to a set of agreed fundholding objectives.

This earlier phase, although only applicable to GPFH, was seen as an important step forward in the quality debate. The authority identified a series of issues for which the first step was the development, with input from local fundholders, of 'best practice templates'. The areas for focus were:

- prescribing policy and practice

- evaluation of services development (and the existing service portfolio)

- business planning, including development of commissioning plans

- teamwork and communication within the practice in relation to fundholding and effective fund management

- clinical audit

- waiting list management

- referral policy and criteria

- monitoring financial performance.

Developing the clinical audit template reportedly proved too difficult at the time, but a draft template was, at the time of the survey, awaiting validation and agreement by the MAAG.

The templates defined standards of practice as:

- excellence in performance

- good performance

- reasonable performance

- the minimum acceptable standards

- performance which falls below a minimum standard of practice.

Following development of the templates and agreement by GPFH representatives, a benchmarking workbook was prepared and disseminated for self-assessment and completion by the fundholders. Whilst there was external involvement (a private consultancy group) in the process, it is interesting to note that self-administration was again the preferred way to assess compliance. The data from the survey were then analysed by Moores Rowland Consulting, and reports prepared for the HA and for the fundholders.

The responses from individual practices were not, however, available to the authority (which, in turn, meant that compliance with standards could not be determined from outside the practice), although each practice was given the data on its relative position vis-à-vis the group as a whole for each of the standards. This programme was not without its problems, since the HA commented that 'progress on this [the priorities for development and programme for implementation] stalled, with a less than lukewarm response from GP fundholders'. However, one mechanism which may stimulate the quality development programme is the involvement of all GPs in the process and, more recently, with the end of GPFH and the development of PCGs, a district-wide programme for assessing quality in primary care has been promoted. The use of benchmarking as a tool to assess the comparative quality of general practice is becoming more widespread, particularly with the expansion of the benchmarking club (*see* Box 5.1) and the lessons that can be learnt from this.

Quality in practice (Solihull HA)

Within Solihull HA, a '*Quality in practice initiative*' has been introduced. A set of local standards has been developed, against which participating practices assess themselves and then submit their assessment for validation. Compliance with the standards is assessed by a team from the HA.

> *The scheme, which is voluntary, is designed to assess practices on the basis of their performance in meeting a set of standards and 'accrediting' the practice in relation to this assessment. The standards devised . . . are consistent with initiatives such as BS 5750, but practices do not need to make a large financial outlay to participate. The initiative started in 1994 . . . and a total of 10 practices have participated to date. (1998 figures)*

The original aims of the Solihull scheme were to:

- ensure that all members of the primary healthcare team are committed to developing quality services and meeting the needs of their local population, through striving continually to improve all aspects of their practice

- develop a PHCT which is strongly motivated to promote, within available resources, excellence in service provision in line with the approach taken in the Patient's Charter.

Literature circulated about the scheme suggests that practices should undertake a detailed preparatory stage in which they consider which of the standards can be satisfied. 'Often a SWOT . . . type analysis can be helpful – but this is at the discretion of the practice. What is important is that the practice consider together how they operate'. There are a number of advantages to such a combined analysis:

- It provides an opportunity to see if the prerequisites for meeting the standards required for the locality scheme are in place, namely:
  - full commitment and leadership from the partners
  - a positive organisational culture with an agreed philosophy for practice, based on shared views which are understood by all staff and to which they show commitment.

- It enables a practice to increase self-knowledge.

Practices are offered guidance/facilitation on undertaking an analysis if this is requested. Having submitted their application, the practice are assessed by a team from the HA who visit the practice to discuss the application made. The team submit a report to the HA, proposing the level of accreditation to be given. Completion of each of the (nine) commitment standards will give the practice a 'credit' (i.e. a maximum of nine credits can be achieved) and according to the number of credits achieved, the practice will receive monies from a non-recurring quality development fund. Under normal circumstances, practices will be expected to meet all the criteria in each standard to gain a credit.

Such an approach was based upon South Derbyshire's *'Commitments to quality'* initiative and the *'Total quality in general practice'* initiative of Hereford and Worcester. The methodology adopted by Solihull represents a form of local 'accreditation' or 'external review' since compliance with local standards and assessment from outside the practice form integral components of the scheme.

Promoting quality in general practice: Bedfordshire HA

Bedfordshire HA has also utilised 'externally developed' assessment tools in the monitoring and improvement of its local primary care services. Whilst there are a number of well-known national models for assessing and monitoring the organisational quality of a practice (KFOA for example), Bedfordshire HA has launched a number of local initiatives to help practices to develop the quality of their services. Their local quality framework has the support of local GPs, practice managers and nurses, and was loosely based on the KFOA programme. It is a self-assessment tool for practices to work with at their own pace. The framework uses an incremental approach:

- Section I deals with essential standards which practices must meet to comply with employment law, health and safety requirements and patients' rights.

- Section II contains basic good practice standards which a number of practices will already be meeting.

- Section III contains desirable standards which practices may choose to aspire to.

The standards cover five main areas of work: provision of services and patient care, health and safety, health records, practice organisation and management and minor surgery. Section I has been available to practices on a voluntary basis since February 1996, and according to the HA more than 60% of practices are already working on the standards contained in it. Dedicated resources were been made available to enable this work to take place.

Additionally, Bedfordshire HA have also promoted the use of development plans, with every practice being required to produce such a three-year plan from 1997/98. This has been perceived as essential to 'strengthening the planning process within the HA . . . and all decisions about investment in individual practices will be based on their plan, and on the overall objectives for the development of services for the locality'. Self-assessment activities, such as the quality framework and clinical audit, will have an important part to play in shaping the business plans. The HA facilitates self-assessment by developing profiling information concerning activity and performance within a practice. This work has already started but will be refined and expanded to enable a practice to have accessible information to allow comparison with other practices.

'Goals for 2000' (East Kent)

The link between business development and investment is not unusual. East Kent, for example, have developed a 'Goals for 2000' strategy, containing standards for non-clinical elements of general practice. Under this scheme, practices are visited once a year by members of the HA's Healthcare Development Department and practice profiles are compiled following such visits. These profiles help inform the development needs of each practice and the HA has committed funding to support practice development in those areas covered by the 'Goals for 2000' standards. Similarly, Lambeth, Southwark and Lewisham HA link resource allocation to the banding of practices under their practice staffing support fund and development policy.

HA accreditation schemes

Northumberland HA

Northumberland HA, in conjunction with Northumberland LMC, have introduced a practice accreditation programme to develop the principles of national accreditation programmes in a local framework. Within Northumberland, a high proportion of practices has participated in the national KFOA programme for primary care, and the HA indicated that the remaining practices agreed to undertake some form of internal review. In total, at the time of the study, 96% of practices had completed the Northumberland practice accreditation programme. The overall aim of the Northumberland scheme has been to improve the organisation of primary healthcare teams to deliver a better level of patient care and the objectives of participation in practice accreditation have been to:

- compare organisational performance against standards

- improve practice organisation

- achieve good patient care

- establish guidelines and protocols

- demonstrate commitment to quality

- identify good practice

- promote educational development.

The 'same standards were set for each practice, enabling all Northumberland practices to assess their performance against each other. It was hoped that the result of this would be improvement of all practices, albeit at a different pace . . . moving towards the same goal . . . it was agreed that there should be five essential standards' to which each Northumberland practice should aspire:

1 Access to surgery consultation.
2 Complaints system.
3 Handling and storage of results.
4 Team meetings.
5 Records management.

Each standard is described by a set of service elements (which detail the purpose of the service) and a set of service descriptions (against which the service can be measured). Criteria are provided for reviewing the extent of compliance with the standards, most of which can be ascertained by a 'yes/no' response. The criteria are arranged hierarchically, further questions demonstrating higher levels of compliance with the standard.

Such standards highlight that, as with many other quality in primary care schemes currently in progress, it is largely the organisation of the practice, as opposed to the outcomes of care or professional competencies, that are the focus of this programme.

Although assessment within the Northumberland accreditation system was that of self-assessment, verification of the results was undertaken by the HA through a visit. This scheme goes beyond many of the other local practice quality initiatives in a number of ways. Firstly, the standards are uniform to all practices in Northumberland (as opposed to being devised by individual practices) and secondly, although initial assessment is from within the practice, further verification/inspection is undertaken by the HA. Additionally, within Northumberland, the visiting team included HA staff who were themselves external surveyors for the KFOA and who therefore had experience outside of a local context. A total of 39 commendations have been given under the scheme, and in areas of exceptional good practice. The review process highlighted a total of 111 recommendations for specific areas of improvement (within all standard categories).

In developing and implementing a local programme of quality development, Northumberland HA are explicit in the problems that they encountered. During the programme there were considerable practical problems experienced in supporting those practices who had demonstrated or identified need, and the HA comment on the fact that the whole process was:

> *inevitably delayed or difficult to implement through lack of appropriate human resources and co-ordination of practical support . . . the needs identified through recommendations far outstripped the support offered.*

In strengthening the local accreditation programme, North-umberland HA are seeking to:

• extend the practice accreditation tool with further standards and criteria which take into account suggestions from practices and include clinical, pharmaceutical and commissioning standards

• set up task groups for developing future standards

• identify resources to support the on-going needs of practices, e.g. manager mentorship

• ensure a multidisciplinary approach to the verification process

• implement a review system for practices which assesses action taken on recommendations.

Personal surveyor experience of national accreditation programmes (KFOA) was utilised by Northumberland HA in its quality development programme for primary care. The existence and availability of such schemes – KFOA (new HQS) and the health services accreditation programme for primary care – was mentioned by a number of HAs in the information that they supplied, although very few indicated how many practices within their district had participated in such programmes. Whereas HAs appeared keen to include all practices in their local programmes for practice development (albeit 'voluntarily'), participation in the more formal, national programmes was seen to arise largely as a result of the 'natural enthusiasm of the practices' – as opposed to being HA driven. There is a clear push for programmes of quality development which have a local focus, are cheaper and which have a high degree of local 'ownership'.

Sheffield HA and Leicestershire HA

An exception to this was the initiative by two HAs within the Trent Region who had looked towards the national programmes for accreditation in primary care when developing their own assessment schemes – although even here local ownership, development and implementation were seen as crucial. Moving towards the more formal model of national accreditation, Sheffield and Leicestershire HAs have sought to involve the majority of practices in an accreditation programme developed in conjunction with the King's Fund and recognised by them. In Sheffield the programme is known as 'Commitment to Quality' (CTQ) and in Leicestershire as 'Blueprint' (BP). Both HAs were concerned to develop a new approach which:

- was attractive to the majority of PHCT

- was based on standards of good practice in primary care developed and owned locally but recognised nationally by an established accrediting body

- encouraged mutual support between PHCTs in developing their plans

- was managed by a HA and encouraged collaborative working with PHCTs

- was more affordable than some of the national initiatives currently available

- would build on and develop the experience and expertise within practices and the HA.

The authorities agreed an approach which would enable PHCTs to improve their performance through:

- a process of review against standards of good practice (which are agreed locally but have national recognition through the King's Fund)

- the development of an action plan to address areas where progress needs to be made

- assessment by healthcare professionals to confirm compliance.

A local steering group was set up to manage, develop and promote the project (with representatives drawn from, amongst others, the HA, PHCTs, MAAG, CHCs and Sheffield RCGP Faculty).

CTQ, in common with other organisational development programmes, seeks to improve the capacity of the whole team to deliver a better service. It is anticipated that participating practices will benefit in the following ways:

- Improved quality, service delivery, organisational culture and structure.

- More effective and efficient working.

- Improved communications.

- Allows the practice to make a public statement on the quality of service.

- CTQ links to other accreditation programmes.

- In the future, participation in quality initiatives may help to secure external funds.

Within the CTQ programme, the King's Fund has undertaken to:

- train facilitators and assessors from Sheffield and Leicestershire

- be involved in final assessment management

- attend a sample of assessments for 'quality assurance' purposes

- approve CTQ under the KFOA programme.

Under the scheme, assessment of Sheffield practices is undertaken by Leicestershire assessors, and vice versa. (Before being accepted as assessors, prospective candidates attend a two-day selection and training event where they are assessed for the skills they need to be effective assessors.) Similar to the higher education models of quality assurance currently run by the Higher Education Funding Council to assess the quality of courses run by HE institutions, the process of assessment involves the writing and collation of documentation prior to the assessment visit, with the visit itself having a number of distinct phases as shown in Table 5.1.

The CTQ standards (Table 5.2) cover four main areas: practice management, team development, clinical effectiveness

Table 5.1   The assessment process

Process of assessment	Timescale	Aspects reviewed
Informal **pre-assessment visit** by own HA/facilitator		• All aspects of assessment covered; brief report from this given to assessors
Pre-assessment documentation	Given to assessment team six weeks prior to visit	• Primary healthcare team profile
		• Practice annual report and practice leaflet
Assessment visit		
Evidence of standards assessment	Reviewed on day	Information relating to standards of care: • Practice plans • Policies, procedures and protocols • Minutes from meeting • Information • Appointments • Personnel records and health records • Professional structures
• Interviews with representatives of staff groups	Reviewed on day	
• Review of patient records	Reviewed on day	
• Review by assessment team	Day of assessment	
• Feedback to practice	Day of assessment	

and prescribing, and under each broad category a number of key issues are considered. Once practices have been assessed and a satisfactory assessment report has been completed, they are fully accredited into the commitment to quality programme for a period of three years. An award certificate and a plaque with the King's Fund logo and the Sheffield Health seal of approval are conferred for the three-year period. After this, practices have to undergo re-inspection to maintain their recognition under the scheme.

Table 5.2 CTQ standards (Sheffield)

Practice management	Team development	Clinical effectiveness	Prescribing
• Annual development plan • Access to services • Involving patients • Information for patients • Complaints • Management of records • Administrative audit • Child protection • Carers • Information management and technology • Financial management • Health and safety • Security of premises • Premises and equipment • Written procedures • Partnership agreement	• Recruitment and selection • Induction and orientation • Staffing arrangements • Education and training • Communication and teamwork • Communication and teamwork – nursing	• Manual of clinical guidelines • Management of asthma • Management of diabetes • Management of coronary heart disease • Management of other diseases • Management of chronic heart failure • Management of hypertension • Stroke prevention • Management of upper GI disorders • Management of epilepsy • Management of back pain • Management of STD • Mental health and social care • Management of enduring mental illness • Management of drug and alcohol misuse • Management of depression • Palliative care	• Quality of prescribing • Repeat prescribing • Generic prescribing • Management of medicines

Table 5.2   (*cont.*)

Practice management	Team development	Clinical effectiveness	Prescribing
		• Child health promotion and immunisation	
		• Consultation times	
		• Continence care	
		• Health record content	
		• Referrals	
		• Clinical audit	
		• Cervical cytology	
		• Management of dementia	
		• Wound care	
		• Maternity care	

Within Sheffield, those practices and individuals participating in the scheme can apply for a small grant (£700 per practice) to cover costs incurred, and PGEA approval for the commitment to quality programme has been given. In Leicestershire, the HA are covering GP locum fees and some additional staff hours (up to £500 GP locum cover and up to four days' staff time for one staff on a claim basis).

For practices who are not yet at a stage to undergo full inspection under the CTQ scheme, the HA is working on a 'credit scheme' whereby practices can focus on and work towards certain standards, and build up credits gradually, eventually leading to full recognition as a CTQ practice. Should practices who successfully complete the CTQ programme wish to continue with another organisational development programme, certain exemptions from the KFOA apply.

The standards for the BP scheme are not as extensive as those for the CTQ, as Table 5.3 illustrates.

To date, only a relatively small number of practices have gone through the CTQ and BP schemes, although commitment to the

Table 5.3   BP standards (Leicestershire)

Practice management	Team development	Organisational development	Policies/procedures etc.
• Practice development plan • Practice charter standards • Staffing arrangements • Information management and technology • Security of systems and premises • Audit • Health records • Health and safety	• Education/ training plan • Appraisal systems • Written job descriptions • Team communication • Audit	• Carers • Serious untoward incidents • Practice leaflet • Complaints/ suggestions procedures	• Health records maintenance • Terminally ill/ bereaved • Child health/ immunisations • Chronic disease management

programmes is strong in each area (from within both the HA and amongst GPs). An evaluation of the accreditation programmes currently running in Sheffield and Leicestershire was undertaken by the HA, in conjunction with the Centre for Health Planning and Management at Keele University.

Other local initiatives

1 Within the West Midlands a number of programmes have developed, many of which have run for some considerable time. In 1991, for example, Hereford and Worcester FHSA initiated a project with local GPs to develop a 'Total quality initiative'. Working with outside consultants, four practices underwent an independent consumer survey and what was termed a 'health check' to determine their strengths and weaknesses. This approach later became the basis for helping practices to implement the Patient's Charter standards.

The emphasis of the documentation assumes that total quality has two main threads:

• Quality in management standards.

• Quality in setting standards for the services provided.

The implementation of the Patient's Charter for GPs is voluntary. The guidance recommends the development of local charters, although it is suggested that these will be more coherent if they are produced by the primary healthcare team rather than by practice staff in isolation. This approach is based upon the expectation that each practice will develop its own standards through analysing its own results and structures. Practices are asked to define how they process patients – the 'quality chain' – and then to identify the key areas for assessing results, specifying the minimum standards in each area and agreeing programme targets for standards above the minimum.

2 The use of statistical packages has increased with the move to closely assess general practice performance. The Isle of Wight HA utilise a range of formal and informal monitoring services (e.g. annual review meetings), and have improved comparative practice profile information by using a computerised performance indicator package developed by their Director of Public Health. This covers a range of quantitative indices and is primarily for use in practices to scrutinise and question any differences perceived between themselves and others. Similarly, a number of HAs have introduced a computerised review package (LAPIS) which enables comparative, systematic assessment across the broad range of services provided within general practice (e.g. Sheffield).

3 Both Lincolnshire Health and Dorset HA are further examples of how strategies and methodologies are being developed and utilised in order to get a handle on quality issues within general practice. Dorset HA has, for example, introduced minimum standards for practice *staff* across all practices in Dorset. The minimum standards relate to reception and administrative staff, practice nursing staff,

dispensers in general practice and practice managers. For practices not attaining these standards, and for those wishing to increase their levels of competency, a training programme has been developed to meet the needs of staff. This includes in-house training for those nurses new to practice nursing, a clinical supervisors' programme, an advisor/mentor programme and development of NVQ 2–5. The 'BTEC Dispensers in General Practice' is also offered.

Additionally, some practices within Dorset have been involved in an organisational development programme, whereby they have been encouraged to consider the systems and structures which need to be in place in order to support high-quality patient care. Like the Northamptonshire approach, the focus within Dorset has been that of organisation, on the premise that 'if a sound organisational base can be achieved, those with the responsibility for the delivery of care are free to concentrate on the high quality of that care'. The organisational development programme was based on principles applied to standards specified by the King's Fund and Dearden Management, with a modular design which could be adapted across practices to meet individual needs.

4 Sandwell HA have extended their 'Good practice' initiative scheme to include innovation in primary care. The scheme was originally developed for secondary care, 'as an alternative to financial penalties and incentives within contracts [and] was . . . based on the idea of encouraging employees to implement changes in practice to improve quality'. In 1997/98, £40 000 of non-recurrent money was set aside to reward good practice initiatives and *all* providers and contractors within Sandwell were invited to submit an application for these awards. Applications were assessed by a panel of judges and 33 awards were made under the scheme (from an entry of 67). The awards are not intended to support the initiatives, rather through recognising the value of such schemes to the community and through widespread publicity and dissemination the benefits are seen to lie in the sharing of

best practice, in staff motivation and in demonstrating the HA's commitment to quality.

The schemes outlined above are illustrative examples. Many other HAs had similar approaches and were working across the authority to develop the quality of GP-based primary care.

Standards and indicators for practice-based care

In common with the local strategies used to determine *individual* performance, the study highlighted that the use of standards and indicators against which to evaluate the quality of *practice-based* services formed a significant area of HA activity: 56 HAs specifically mentioned that their use formed a major topic for working group discussions; and 49 reported that they used some form of locally derived indicator(s) to assess the quality of practice-based care. Dorset HA had, at the time of the study,

> *recently undertaken several pieces of work in identifying practices who may be perceived as under-performing in certain areas, and has been working closely with all practices in determining indicators of good practice. A variety of comparative indicators have been developed which compare practices' performance in general medical services, prescribing and secondary care utilisation. With the exception of prescribing, practice values are compared to the Dorset average and a local average (i.e. comparing practices with other practices in the same locality) . . . Further links between the indicators are being developed.*

A survey by Campbell *et al.* (1997) identified that a number of quality indicators were being developed and used by HAs, and:

> *. . . although only a 43% response rate was achieved, the survey highlighted that indicators were most commonly being used in the areas of access, organisational aspects of*

Technical	Interpersonal

Structure

Direct—inspection

```
        ┌ Facilities*
        │ Team*
      ─ │ Clinics*
        │ Protocols*
        │ Premises*
Indirect—questionnaire* └ Procedures*
```

```
Interview/
questionnaire*      ─
e.g. PPG brochure*
```

```
┌ Attitudes
│ Beliefs
│ Availability*
│ Amenities*
│ Patient liaison*
└ Inspection*
```

Process

```
                      ┌ Sit in
           ┌ Direct ⟨─ Audio tape
Observation ─           └ Video tape
           │           Records*
           └ Indirect  Patients
```

```
                       ┌ Sit in
            ┌ Direct ⟨ Audio tape
Observation ─            Video tape
            └ Indirect ─ Satisfaction
                         scales
```

Prescribing (i.e. generic prescribing rates)

Outcome

Prescribing (appropriate prescribing practice)

Intermediate   Screening/**Prevention***

```
        ┌────┬────┐
        BP  Smears* Immunisations*
```

```
        ┌ Problem outcome
Final ⟨── Mortality
        └ Specific studies (key cases/
                            conditions)
```

```
           ┌ Satisfaction/
           │ complaints
Patients ⟨── Compliance
           └ Behaviour
```

Key:

* = commonly cited areas where HA standards and indicators have been developed to
    assess the provision of GP-based services.
    Figure adapted from Baker (1992).

Figure 5.1   Standards and indicators for general practice.

care, preventative care, care for a small number of chronic diseases, prescribing and gate-keeping. No identified indicators related to effective communication, care for acute illness, health outcomes or patient evaluation.

The current study reviewed the range and type of indicators that were being used by HAs. Despite the national emphasis on outcomes, a large proportion of standards and indicators still focuses on the contextual or process aspects of care provision, rather than looking at the direct professional/patient interaction or detailed outcomes for specific treatments. Additionally, many HAs needed to exercise caution when using the terms 'standard' and 'indicator', since there was a clear lack of comprehension about the differences between the two.

The one exception to the emphasis on the contextual delivery of care is the widespread use of prescribing indicators for assessing the quality of care provided both at an individual practitioner level and, through aggregation, at a practice and HA level. Anomalous prescribing has both professional, health-related and financial implications, and managing prescribing budgets and ensuring high-quality practice within this sphere are well-documented areas of concern.

However, whilst prescribing indicators were commonly used as 'quality' indicators, there were limitations of the data available to accurately assess prescribing practices:

> . . . there are serious limitations to the use of [Prescription Pricing Authority] data to assess quality of prescribing, as much of the clinical background has to be inferred and even quantities prescribed for patients can only be estimated or obtained by specific manual searches at the PPA. Much discussion takes place with GPs around cost effectiveness in prescribing, but opinion varies greatly in the quality vs. cost arguments which take place (North Staffordshire HA).

Furthermore, in a study of 115 HAs and health commissions, Baker (1996) found that:

> . . . some [prescribing] indicators were based on the idiosyncratic view of a local pharmaceutical or medical adviser. In other areas considerable efforts had gone into involving general practitioners in consensus groups to produce indicators in prescribing agreeable to all concerned. Respondents also reported great variation in the application of indicators: some were using them to highlight areas of

prescribing that needed further discussion with the practice, while others were tying them to resource allocation measures . . . the derivation and application of prescribing indicators vary widely.

Consequently, whilst a range of indicators may be utilised by HAs in their attempts to determine the quality of primary care, such indicators are not necessarily representative of good practice or high-quality service provision. Rather, as with the indicator sets used to assess individual performance, more rigorous development is required relating to their focus, maturation, implementation and relationship to each other. Although a number of HAs emphasised the need to move towards developing clinical indicators, for the majority this is still some way off.

Achieving a consensus concerning 'good practice' in the organisational and managerial aspects of care has taken considerable time and effort, and the prospect of introducing clinical and outcome measures for general practice requires yet more investment. However, with PCGs required to show measurable improvements in the health of local populations, standards and indicators which relate to the actual delivery of services and the impact of care will *have* to play an increasing role in assessments of quality and performance in general practice. Attention must be given to the key issues which follow.

Key issues in the management of quality and performance in general practice

HAs have clearly put considerable efforts into promoting quality within general practice. There are, however, a number of aspects which need to be addressed when looking at how quality and performance are managed both within general practice and in the wider healthcare arena.

1 Developing a common approach to quality assessment

Significant differences exist when looking at the various HA schemes developed to address aspects of quality and performance in general practice (*see* Box 5.2).

This poses a number of problems when seeking to promote equity within the NHS and to ensure, at the very least, a baseline standard of service provision within general practice. The introduction of clinical governance and PCGs further complicates matters. Not only will pre-existing initiatives need to be located within a wider, more coherent and comprehensive performance management and accountability framework but the whole question of who is responsible for developing and assessing quality and performance in general practice has become more complex.

There is also a need to develop a clear view of quality (possibly across several dimensions – personal/professional/organisational/ user, etc.) and how this will be managed and developed.

HAs have a particular view regarding quality and performance management, which has been applied to general practice throughout an area. The advent of PCGs and PCTs may lead to greater variation in the performance management process:

> *each organisation will have to learn how to define and determine quality . . . the appropriate orientation for the standards will be determined by the operations of the PCGs which will require an analysis of their organisational form.*
> (Scrivens 1998)

With PCGs consisting of multidisciplinary teams (who may have little history of working together), achieving a consensus about quality management could prove problematic. In addition, each professional group (medical, managerial, professions allied to medicine) may have competing priorities which could hinder attempts to implement new procedures in line with central

Box 5.2: Developing quality in general practice: the range of standards and methods of validation

- High degree of formality and external validation, i.e. formal, national accreditation programmes.

- Practices involved in national programme. Assessed by external agency. Indicators used are perceived as nationally agreed targets for good practice. Comparability possible within and between HAs. Compliance leads to nationally recognised award.

- Practices actively involved in utilising nationally devised programme of quality assurance at a local level. Assessed by team of HA staff and other professionals. Compliance may result in a locally recognised award.

- Practices participate in locally devised programme of quality assurance. Practices assess their own performance against a set of locally agreed standards and this is then verified by an outside agency (i.e. validated by non-HA staff). Compliance may result in a locally recognised award.

- Practices involved in locally devised programme of quality assurance. Practices assess their own performance against a set of locally agreed standards, and their performance is then assessed by HA staff (i.e. externally validated). Compliance with the standards may result in a locally recognised award.

- Practices are actively involved in locally devised programme of quality assurance. Practices set their own standards and assess their own performance. This is then externally validated by peers/HA.

- Practices actively involved in locally devised programme of quality assurance. Practices assess their own performance against a set of locally agreed standards, which is then summarised and sent to the HA.

- Practices actively involved in locally devised programme of quality assurance. Practices set own standards, and assess their own performance. Minimum criteria typically apply.

- Practices aware of quality assurance through work of HA. Practices draw up plans to assess current performance and future development.

- A range of quality measures in use (i.e. ad hoc surveys, reviews of complaints, practice visits). Little developmental or strategic work regarding the quality of services on offer.

- Low formality/little strategic direction.

policy. As was alluded to earlier, although national policy gives a definition of quality, putting this into practice (i.e. determining what is 'right') may not be the easiest of tasks.

2 A multidimensional approach

To date, the composition of many performance working groups has been heavily biased towards medical representatives (for the reasons suggested earlier). The new performance management agenda calls for all those involved in the care process, together with patients themselves, to have a major role in determining the quality of service provision. Giving equal weight to user views – particularly when seen in the context of their exclusion from many of the quality schemes developed by HAs – will undoubtedly take time.

3 Greater appreciation of the advantages and limits of the methodologies used to assess quality and performance

The range of methodologies currently in use (*see* Box 5.2) emphasises that some groups prefer internally developed and assessed quality schemes, whilst others seek to demonstrate achievement of national standards of care through external review. Whichever method is preferred, the reasons for choosing a particular approach must be clearly stated and the advantages and limitations appreciated. PCGs and HAs also need to have clear definitions concerning the standards and indicators that they use to assess care provision. The current situation, with little terminological distinction, can only be a recipe for confusion. As Scrivens (1998) notes:

> the content of the various [quality] models is difficult to analyse . . . because those developing the concepts are tending to move between a number of different theoretical frames. For example, management functions are described as performance dimensions, performance is confused both

with the concept of quality and the measurement of quality and tools for promoting good performance. There is a need for a more consistent vocabulary and theoretical framework.

4 Health economics, the cost of (poor) quality and opportunities missed

Only a very small minority of HAs stated that economic evaluations formed part of their approach to service planning and delivery, yet inappropriate care, however defined, can be costly in both monetary and personal terms. The costs of implementing the new procedures were frequently cited as a barrier to progress, yet this was not accompanied by an assessment of the relative costs of poor quality care (since the 'consequential costs' may be borne by another party or are less easily discernible). With the requirement to demonstrate 'efficiency' and 'effectiveness' high on the health agenda, HAs and PCGs cannot ignore the role of health economics in assessing and developing local services.

5 Performance – effecting change through support

The new performance management procedures should be 'inclusive . . . reflective and supportive for doctors, nurses and other health professionals' (Health Service Circular 1998/139). This raises questions about how professional performance is appraised, particularly within organisations experiencing both widespread and rapid change. The whole question of performance assessment and attribution needs to be handled in a sensitive manner, since individuals (and collective groups) may put up barriers when they feel under 'threat'. Effective partnerships and the notion of 'trust' between all those involved were seen as key factors in progressing this particular issue. However, the challenges posed by the restructuring of primary care clearly affected both the culture and the working relationships between the various professionals and organisations concerned.

6 Appropriate data

Whilst many HAs had clearly moved forward in developing new performance management systems, there was a widespread belief that the inaccuracies or inadequacies of the data available prevented more detailed assessments of provision. This was particularly so when discussing clinical aspects of the care process and outcome measurements. As one HA director recently commented 'we simply don't know what general practitioners are doing . . . we have no notion of what clinical competence is, so how can we monitor and improve it?' (Marshall 1999). With the need to demonstrate continuous quality improvement – 'achievable change, with a focus on specific issues' (HSC 1998/ 139) – data will be required not only to show that an organisation is meeting the requirements of the clinical governance agenda, but also to assess the impact of any quality improvement or performance management programme. This calls for longitudinal, comparative programmes of assessment at practitioner, patient, practice and population levels (Poole 1999).

7 Developing quality within an overall strategy for service development

It is essential for each PCG (or care provider) to have a strategic plan for service provision and service development. This should contain key objectives which relate to the standard or quality of care provided, as opposed to simply specifying that a particular service area will be developed – although very few of the HAs taking part in the survey outlined explicit objectives for GP-based care. With the development of accountability agreements under clinical governance, the impact of PCG plans on performance across the six areas of the NHS performance assessment framework (i.e. health improvement, fair access, effective delivery of appropriate healthcare, efficiency, patient/carer experience, health outcomes) will be reviewed. The NHS long-term service agreements will also enable a more rigorous form of performance review to be undertaken.

8 Ensuring that quality is assessed across the organisation

The costs of developing and implementing new procedures and of supporting remedial action could lead to HAs and PCGs concentrating on key strategic or policy-led areas as opposed to developing an integrated approach to quality development across the organisation.

9 Developing appropriate methodologies to evaluate primary care

Primary care is distinguished by a variety of organisational forms and professional inter-relationships. Therefore, any *organisationally* based quality approach, such as the accreditation philosophies and schemes introduced to assess the provision of hospital-based care, will either have to force the development of a manageable hierarchical organisational structure or will have to be adapted to reflect an alternative perception of organisational structure. The latter requires a more collective, participative and, arguably, to some extent, a professionally dominated model of organisation (Scrivens and Blaylock 1997).

10 Role clarification

With PCGs bringing together a wide range of individuals and groups, and with the role of the HA changed following the introduction of PCGs, it is likely that the roles and responsibilities of those within both organisations will take time to become re-established. Managing performance assessment programmes and effecting change during such transitionary periods may therefore prove difficult. Implementing clinical governance requires strong leadership and political and personal sensitivity when dealing with both individuals and collective interest groups.

11 Appropriate targeting

In developing quality strategies and systems, a major consideration has to be that of appropriate targeting. That is to say, are strategies, standards and procedures developed which identify those practices or individuals who provide care which is at the 'trailing' edge of acceptable performance, or are standards and indicators developed which promote high-quality practice? This is a significant question, since the approaches and methodologies are not the same and one has to ask which approach is likely to yield maximum benefit in terms of improving the overall quality of primary care services provision.

12 Impact evaluations

There is currently a lack of data concerning the progress of the various schemes targeted at GP performance or at developing quality in general practice. Accordingly, it has been difficult to assess the impact of such programmes and the barriers to progress and change are only now becoming transparent (Birch and Scrivens 1999; Marshall 1999).

Summary

In 1996, the Shields Report in Scotland emphasised that 'greater external peer review of NHS provision of all services is required'. They also noted that whilst 'formal national accreditation systems were unlikely to be the answer to monitoring quality, local accreditation-type systems may well be a popular solution'. This would indeed appear to be the case, since the majority of HAs appear to favour locally derived systems of review. Whilst there is a growing recognition of the need to look towards a more standard-ised framework for quality assessment, reflective of the move to introduce national performance indicators, the current situation, with a myriad of different schemes and methodologies highlights that there is still much work to be done to achieve this goal.

With the confusion over appropriate methodologies and the need to develop reliable and valid clinical and non-clinical measures to assess the quality of care, it is apparent that there is no short-term solution to the issue of performance monitoring. Nonetheless, salient lessons can be learnt from those HAs who are advanced in their procedures and from the national organisations who seek to demonstrate good practice throughout the NHS.

With the quality of NHS care firmly established on the policy agenda, the key issues surrounding performance assessment and quality development cannot be ignored in the long-term. It is clear, for example, that:

> the NHS can expect continued attention to measured indicators of performance in the context of national comparisons. (Davies and Lampel 1998)

HAs, PCGs and PCTs must strive to create an environment that enables the quality of service provision to be improved across the board – but they cannot do it in isolation. They need to work together, and with the professions involved and other interested parties, to achieve this aim.

Chapter 6

Developing clinical governance in primary care

As the review of performance management procedures has demonstrated, considerable attention has been given over a long period of time to issues concerning the assessment of individual and organisational quality. However, with the introduction of clinical governance, all NHS organisations will have to review their entire approach towards quality and performance assessment. All performance-related initiatives[1] will have to be documented, and located within an overarching framework which illustrates that an organisation is managing performance and looking to improve quality across the board.

With changing patterns of healthcare delivery and a blurring of the boundaries between service providers, it is necessary for HAs, PCGs and PCTs to consider the totality of NHS care and how the many activities which support performance management and quality in healthcare can be located within a system-wide view of clinical governance. This chapter outlines the key components of clinical governance and presents a model which sites the differing

---

[1] These include, *inter alia*, professional assessments, in-house quality review schemes, assessments by other agencies (i.e. Health and Safety), risk management, clinical audit, user feedback.

activities undertaken within primary care into a coherent and systematic framework.

Clinical governance[2]

Despite widespread support for the general principles of clinical governance (Scrivens 1998), developing a framework for it and establishing a working model present considerable challenges. Clinical governance has been defined as:

> *a system through which NHS organisations are accountable for continuously improving the quality of their services and safeguarding high standards of care by creating an environment in which excellence in clinical care will flourish.* (DoH 1999c)

This places clinical governance as an approach to *managing* quality of healthcare services and as such it requires a framework within which successful management can occur.

Translating the concept of clinical governance into practice therefore requires:

- structures through which to make the concept meaningful

- tools to create actions

- communication, to ensure that people charged with carrying out the tasks can fully understand appropriate action.

The White Paper (DoH 1997) and the accompanying consultation document, *A First Class Service* (1998a), provide the principles upon which a system of clinical governance can be based. As we have seen, the White Paper espouses a 'right first time' view of

---

[2] This chapter draws on the results of a scoping study commissioned by the Department of Health concerning clinical governance in primary care (Scrivens 1998). The views contained in the report are those of the author and do not reflect the views of the Department of Health.

quality which also emphasises the patient experience and, in line with modern thinking about quality, promotes visible and rigorous management of performance, continuous quality improvement and team working.

> *There will be a 'third way' of running the NHS – a system based on partnership and driven by performance . . .*

> *A new system of clinical governance in NHS Trusts and primary care to ensure that clinical standards are met, and that processes are in place to ensure continuous quality improvement, backed by a new statutory duty for quality in NHS Trusts.*

The White Paper also makes provision for a system of quality assurance of the arrangements for clinical governance through the work of the Commission for Health Improvement.

> *The Commission for Health Improvement will complement the introduction of clinical governance arrangements. As a statutory body at arms length from the Government, the new Commission will offer an independent guarantee that local systems to monitor, assure and improve clinical quality are in place. It will support local developments and 'spot-check' the new arrangements.*

Under the functions of a good organisation it notes that *quality improvement processes* (e.g. clinical audit) should be in place and integrated with the quality programme for the organisation as a whole.

> *Every part of the NHS, and everyone who works in it, should take responsibility for working to improve quality. This must be quality in its broadest sense: doing the right things, at the right time, for the right people and doing them right – first time. And it must be the quality of the patient's experience as well as the clinical result – quality measured*

> *in terms of prompt access, good relationships and efficient administration. (Para 3.2)*

The report also outlines those *organisational functions* which may form the basis for any performance review programme, including:

- leadership
- management of information page
- improving organisational performance
- continuum of care
- education
- a patient focus

and incorporates a number of *performance dimensions* (DoH 1997, 1998b) around which assessment should occur. These are:

- health improvement
- fair access
- effective delivery of appropriate healthcare
- efficiency
- patient/carer experience
- health outcomes.

These six performance dimensions can broadly be restated in service delivery terms as: appropriateness, availability, timeliness, effectiveness, co-ordination of care, safety and risk assessment, efficiency, respect and caring. Whilst a number of these may not be well developed for care provided outside of the acute or hospital environment, they nonetheless offer the basis for the development of a more relevant model for the management of primary care.

A variety of national bodies involved with general practice and primary care (e.g. the GMC, the RCGP, the British Association of Medical Managers, the National Primary Care Research and

Development Centre and the Eli Lilley Centre for Primary Care) have suggested models for implementing clinical governance (e.g. Baker *et al.* 1999). Whilst many of these clearly promote a more consistent approach to performance management within primary care and offer ways in which clinical governance can be addressed, there remains a need for greater terminological distinction and a better appreciation of the new organisational structures within which clinical governance is being applied.

Developing clinical governance within PCGs/PCTs

Both the structure and composition of PCGs (and PCTs) may, in themselves, present problems in advancing the new performance management agenda. As Scrivens (1998) notes:

> *in the context of primary care, where there is no established hierarchical management structure, the implementation of performance management and accountability through management may present difficulties.*

PCGs are what might be described as 'flat' organisations, bringing together groups of GPs and other professionals who may have little history of collaborative working.

Equally, as Scally and Donaldson (1998) demonstrate (albeit unintentionally perhaps), there may be practical difficulties in translating an essentially secondary care view of clinical governance into a primary care context. They state that clinical governance:

> *must be rigorous in its application, organisation-wide in its emphasis, accountable in its delivery, developmental in its thrust and positive in its connotations . . . the development of clinical governance is designed to consolidate, codify, and universalise often fragmented and far from clear policies and approaches, to create organisations in which the final*

> *accountability for clinical governance rests with the chief executive of the health organisation – with regular reports to board meetings – and daily responsibility rests with a senior clinician.*

This is a:

> *set of statements normally associated with a quality assurance approach for a hierarchically structured organisation. They assume therefore a coherent, managed organisation in which individuals and the organisational systems are well defined and capable of hierarchical management.* (Scrivens 1998)

For those involved in the development and operation of PCGs and PCTs, such statements may not fit with either current or future organisational forms.

Recent thinking about performance review processes (as illustrated by the National Framework for Assessing Performance) suggests that the main emphasis should be on performance (expressed through process and outcome indicators) as opposed to looking predominantly at structures and processes. However, not only are there debates around the appropriateness of indicators to assess quality, particularly when thinking of the total package of care, but it is also important that any standards or indicators which relate to the management of quality reflect the maturity of the organisation itself:

> *. . . there are two important lessons that analysts of quality management systems have learnt in the past. The nature of the standards used by organisations to develop quality assurance processes must be selected by the ability of the organisations to deal with the management processes associated with quality. That is, the less mature the organisation in dealing with the management of quality, the more structured the standards must be. **The less the***

experience an organisation has of quality assurance, the more help it needs in establishing its approaches to quality. Although the professional bodies in primary care have considerable experience in the professional determination of quality (although there may be considerable differences between the various perspectives and quality/performance management schemes), the organisations set up to deal with quality issues will be newborn. (Scrivens 1998)

The appropriate orientation for the standards will therefore be determined by the configuration and work of PCGs/PCTs themselves, which in turn requires an analysis of their organisational forms. Given the potential problems of assessing such newly created organisations (primary care has only recently moved away from what might be termed a system of 'networks' to a more integrated organisational format), it is necessary to identify different performance dimensions which can be assessed at every appropriate level.

A proposed model for clinical governance in primary care

As Sections I and II have highlighted that, when reviewing the performance of any organisation there are different dimensions which can be identified, reflecting clinical, managerial and patient concerns. These can, in turn, be related to a series of questions reflecting the performance of the individual or organisation, and a range of methods may be employed to determine the level of compliance or performance against the various dimensions selected. Whilst the majority of HA schemes outlined in Section II were developed *prior* to the introduction of clinical governance, it is possible to see how a similar approach may be utilised when developing a comprehensive and integrated performance management system for clinical governance.

As Table 6.1 illustrates, a number of key areas concerning the performance of any organisation can be outlined. The specific areas listed in the first column, for example, were initially identified in 1995 in the *Joint Commission of Accreditation of Hospitals Manual* as salient measures of performance for hospitals, and these have subsequently been adapted by Scrivens (1998) for the study of performance relating to clinical governance. Having identified the key areas for assessment, it is then possible to consider the range of questions which might be asked to determine performance in these areas and also to consider what methods and data sources could be used to review performance.

It *is* therefore possible for there to be a national framework for performance assessment (i.e. the dimensions outlined in Table 6.1) which does not necessarily dictate the processes used to monitor performance or to achieve it. The emphasis on personal responsibility, for example, suggests that each individual practitioner should be capable of assessing their own performance relative to the key areas; equally each practice, each PCG and each HA should be demonstrating compliance/assessment at each level.

Scrivens (1998) also suggests that one of the key factors in establishing a model or framework for clinical governance relates to how the organisation is structured and managed. For example, the management of primary care organisations – whether they are community pharmacies, general dental practices, general medical practices or primary care teams – typically covers four basic areas:

1 Clinical or technical aspects relating to the ability of the primary care practitioner to provide the most appropriate and efficacious care to individual patients within the limits of resources and current knowledge.
2 The ability of the primary care practitioner to work in partnership with colleagues in other care-providing organisations, such as hospitals, social services and the voluntary sector, to provide continuous clinical and social care for an individual patient across a number of different organisations.

Table 6.1 Clinical governance: dimensions of performance and potential approaches (Scrivens 1998)

Dimensions	Types of questions	Examples of approaches	Review
Efficacy	Are the outcomes those expected?	Clinical audit, guidelines,	Accreditation, PCG peer review, external review HA review by designated officer
Appropriateness	Are the tests the ones expected?	Clinical audit, national standards, guidelines	National and local review processes
Availability	Are the right tests, clinics, services available?	Evidence-based review of practice	Accreditation, PCG peer review, external review HA review by designated officer
Timeliness	Assessment of time to get tests, see patients, etc.?	Audit of time to get tests, etc.	Indicators, benchmarking Internal and external review
Effectiveness	Is care provided in the correct manner?	Adherence to guidelines	National and local review processes
Co-ordination	Is care co-ordinated?	Review of co-ordination of care	Accreditation, PCG peer review, external review HA review by designated officer
Safety	What risk assessments are done?	Risk assessment	Accreditation, PCG peer review, external review HA review by designated officer
Efficiency	Are resources achieving the desired outcomes?	Comparison of outcomes with resources used	Indicators, benchmarking Internal and external review
Respect and caring	How are patients treated?	Patient involved in decisions and patient satisfaction	Accreditation, PCG peer review, external review HA review by designated officer

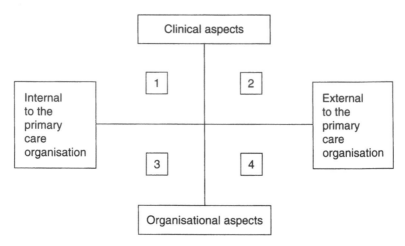

Figure 6.1   A model for clinical governance in primary care (developed by Scrivens 1998).

3   The ability of the primary care organisation to organise its internal resources to ensure that patients are treated speedily, with respect and dignity and provided with appropriate information.

4   The management of resources of the primary care organisation in relation to the local population (availability of care, waiting times, health status) using population-based data.

These areas can also be grouped into clinical aspects of care (both internal and external) internal administration and management, and management of external information and resources which can be placed on two axes as in Figure 6.1. The resulting four quadrants produce the domains of clinical and organisational management which are fundamental to the successful working of any primary care organisation.

- **Domain 1** concerns the clinical activities within primary care – the practitioner/patient encounter. This requires that the right treatment is given in the right way.

- **Domain 2** concerns the relationship of clinical activities with other care agencies and the processes developed to ensure that the right care is given in the right way.

- **Domain 3** concerns the administrative processes used to support the delivery of care and to provide an appropriate environment in which both the effectiveness of care and patient satisfaction can be maximised.

- **Domain 4** concerns the use of externally and internally generated information and communications systems to ensure that resources effectively and efficiently support the clinical and social aspects of care.

Tools exist to support the activities conducted within each of these domains. The following are well-known examples already in use in many parts of primary care:

- Domain 1 can be supported by clinical audit, evidence-based information, diagnostic computer systems, patient information systems, standards-based review systems such as accreditation, RCGP assessment schemes, and patient complaints not only to provide better processes, but also to highlight where the provision of care could be improved. This might lead to changes in systems, programmes of continuing professional development, etc.

- Domain 2 can be supported by care pathways, referral and treatment guidelines. Areas for improvement would be high-lighted by clinical audit, patient complaints, peer review, etc.

- Domain 3 may be supported by standards-based review systems such as accreditation, HA standards, RCGP assessment schemes, the European Foundation for Quality Model, etc. In association with patients' complaints, these can also identify areas for improvement.

- Domain 4 can be supported by population databases, information on waiting lists and waiting times, and other analyses conducted by national benchmarking systems which will highlight areas for improvement.

Clinical governance could ask for a demonstration that tools are being used within each domain to promote the management of

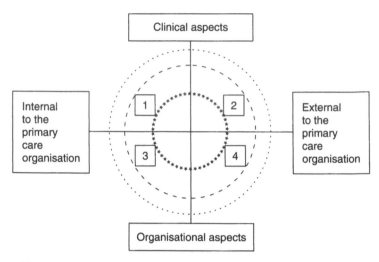

Key: ****** Individual   - - - Team   ·····PCG or other organisation

Figure 6.2   The differing levels of clinical governance activity.

primary care across all of these domains. However, it is possible that a primary care organisation could have all of these things in place but fail to be continuously trying to improve. Therefore, it is necessary to add a requirement that the quadrants are used to demonstrate that continuous efforts to understand performance and to improve are being undertaken.

To make the task of demonstrating continuous improvement easier, it is possible to provide a pro-forma of relevant performance dimensions. For example, if the following performance dimensions are selected – appropriateness, availability, timeliness, effectiveness, co-ordination of care, safety and risk assessment, efficiency, and respect and caring – each primary care organisation can be asked how it is improving by using tools to check on quality and about its thinking regarding improvement in each of these performance dimensions, using the four quadrants of activity as a guide.

It is also important to recognise that clinical governance applies to all tiers within an organisation and should not only look at clinical and non-clinical activity and consider internal and external influences, but should also consider these at the individual, team and PCG level (as shown in Figure 6.2).

Thinking towards the future

Moving the clinical governance agenda forward will require considerable effort, time and resources for PCGs, PCTs and HAs. However, as the review of HA approaches to improving performance in general practice illustrated, it is possible to develop quality programmes which have widespread support from local practitioners. In those HAs where quality and performance management have been placed high on the agenda and where all those involved are working together to try to develop local service provision, the benefits *are* beginning to be felt at a number of levels (Birch and Scrivens 1999; Scrivens *et al.* 2000), although such progress is far from uniform.

It is worth reflecting that those sites where substantial progress has been made exhibit a number of common features. For new initiatives such as clinical governance to be developed and progressed it is imperative that all those within the organisation are working towards a common goal. To achieve this, good dialogue within the organisation is required and working practices need to be both visible and reflective. Equally fundamental is the requirement for any organisation which has undergone significant reorganisation and structural change to establish a clear management and leadership structure with designated responsibilities, and to ensure that the appropriate organisational infrastructure is in place to support the new developments.

It is important not to lose sight of the considerable progress that has been made in the performance management arena, both nationally and locally, and as the review of HA strategies has shown, many of those involved in the quality debate have a clear commitment to improving services and providing high-quality care. Whilst there is undoubtedly a great deal of support for the principles of clinical governance and widespread acceptance that the existing inequalities in health and in service provision need to be ameliorated, whether this can be sustained in the face of future policy developments, service reorganisations and changes in the wider socio-economic environment remains to be seen.

References

Acheson D (1998) *Independent Inquiry into Inequalities in Health.* The Stationery Office, London.

Baker R (1992) *Practice Assessment and Quality of Care.* RCGP, London.

Baker R, Lakhani M, Fraser R and Cheater F (1999) A model for clinical governance in primary care groups. *BMJ.* **318**: 779–83.

Baker S (1996) Use of performance indicators for general practice. *BMJ.* **312**: 58.

Birch K (1997) *Great Expectations: a sociological analysis of women's experiences of maternity care in the 'new' NHS* (PhD thesis). University of Liverpool. Unpublished.

Birch K and Scrivens E (1999) *Developing Indicators for General Practice: a case study.* Centre for Health Planning and Management, Keele University.

Brook RH and Lohr KN (1985) Efficacy, effectiveness, variations and quality: boundary crossing research. *Medical Care* **23**(5): 710–22.

Brooks S (1994) Personal communication.

Campbell SM *et al.* (1997) *Quality Indicators for General Practice: which ones can GPs and health authority managers agree on?* National Primary Care Research and Development Centre, University of Manchester.

Centre for the Evaluation of Public Policy and Practice (1991) *Considering Quality: an analytical guide to the literature on quality standards in the public services.* Brunel University.

Chief Medical Officer (1997) *Annual Report.* The Stationery Office, London.

Daltroy LH and Liang MH (1991) Advances in patient education in rheumatic disease. *Ann Rheum Dis.* **50** (Suppl 3): 415–17.

Davies HTO and Lampel J (1998) Trust in performance indicators. *Quality in Health Care* **7**(3): 159.

Department of Health and Social Security (1980) *Report of the Working Group on Inequalities in Health (Black Report).* HMSO, London.

Department of Health (1989) *Working for Patients.* HMSO, London.

Department of Health (1991) *The Patient's Charter*. HMSO, London.

Department of Health (1996) *Primary Care: delivering the future*. The Stationery Office, London.

Department of Health (1997) *The New NHS: modern, dependable*. The Stationery Office, London.

Department of Health Press Release (20 May 1997) *New Powers for Action Against Inefficient Doctors*.

Department of Health (1998a) *A First Class Service*. The Stationery Office, London.

Department of Health (1998b) *The New NHS: modern, dependable. A National Framework for Assessing Performance*. The Stationery Office, London.

Department of Health (1998c) *Clinical Effectiveness Indicators: a consultation document*. The Stationery Office, London.

Department of Health (1999a) *Steps Towards Clinical Governance*. DoH, Leeds.

Department of Health (1999b) *Our Healthier Nation*. The Stationery Office, London.

Department of Health (1999c) *Supporting Doctors, Protecting Patients: a consultation paper on preventing, recognising and dealing with poor clinical performance of doctors in the NHS in England*. DoH, London.

Donabedian A (1980) The definition of quality: a conceptual exploration. In: *Explorations in Quality Assessment and Monitoring* (vol 1). Health Administration Press, Ann Arbor.

Drummond M, Stoddart G and Torrance G (1987) *Methods for the Economic Evaluation of Health Care Programmes*. Oxford Medical Publications, Oxford.

Fitzpatrick R *et al.* (1984) Satisfaction with health care. In: Fitzpatrick R, Hinton J, Newman S, Scambler G (eds) *The Experience of Illness*. Tavistock, London.

Fry D (1990) Systems of standards for community health services in Australia. *Quality Assurance in Health Care* 2(1): 59–67.

Gilpatrick E (1999) *Quality Improvement Projects in Health Care: problem solving in the workplace*. Sage, London.

Giuffrida A, Gravelle H and Roland M (1999) Measuring quality of care with routine data: avoiding confusion between performance indicators and health outcomes. *BMJ*. **319**: 94–8.

Gray DP (1992) Accreditation in general practice. *Quality in Health Care* 1: 61–4.

Grenville J (1998) Personal communication.

Ham C and Hunter D (1988) *Managing Clinical Acitivity in the NHS*. King's Fund Institute, London.

House of Commons Health Committee (1992) *Report on Maternity Services.* HMSO, London.

Huntington J (1994) GP education bottom of the class. *Health Service Journal* **104**: 22–4.

Hutchinson A (1997) Presentation to Royal College of General Practitioners Conference 14 November 1997, *Measuring General Practice.*

Irvine D (1997) The performance of doctors II. *BMJ.* **314**: 1613–15.

Irvine D (1999a) Dysfunctional doctors: the GMCs new approach. In: Rosenthal MM *et al.* (eds) *Medical Mishaps: pieces of the puzzle.* Open University Press, Buckingham.

Irvine D (1999b) The performance of doctors: the new professionalism. *Lancet* **353**: 1174–7.

Irvine D and Irvine S (1996) *The Practice of Quality.* Radcliffe Medical Press, Oxford.

Joint Commission on Accreditation of Healthcare Organisations (1989) Characteristics of clinical indicators. *Quarterly Review Bulletin* **15**: 330–9.

Joint Commission on Accreditation of Healthcare Organisations (1995) *Agenda for Change: developing an indicator-based monitoring system.* JCAHO.

King's Fund (1996) *Primary Health Care Organisational Audit Manual.* King's Fund, London.

Koch H (1992) *Total Quality Management in Healthcare* Macmillan, Basingstoke.

Leatherman S and Sutherland K (1998) Evolving quality in the new NHS: policy, process and pragmatic considerations. *Quality in Health Care* December supplement: *Organisational Change: the key to quality improvement.*

Majeed F and Voss S (1995) Performance indicators for general practice. *BMJ.* **311**: 209–10.

Marshall M (1999) Improving quality in general practice: qualitative case study of barriers faced by health authorities *BMJ.* **319**: 164–7.

Mason V (1989) *Women's Experiences of Maternity Care: a survey manual.* OPCS, London.

Maxwell RJ (1984) Quality assessment in health care. *BMJ.* **288**: 1470–2.

McColl A, Roderick P, Gabbay J, Smith H and Moore M (1998) Performance indicators for primary care groups: an evidence-based approach. *BMJ.* **317**: 1354–60.

Meads G (1997) Presentation to Royal College of General Practitioners Conference 14 November 1997, *Measuring General Practice.*

Moore R (1996) *The MRCGP Examination.* RCGP, London.

Morgan M, Calnan M and Manning N (1985) *Sociological Approaches to Health and Medicine*. Croom Helm, London.

National Association of Commissioning GPs (1997) *Annual Conference Report*.

Øvretveit J (1993) *Measuring Service Quality*. TQM Practitioner Series, Technical Communications Publishing Ltd, Hertfordshire.

Øvretveit J (1999) *Integrated Quality Development in Public Healthcare: a comparison of six hospitals quality programmes and a practical theory for quality development*. The Norwegian Medical Association, Oslo.

Paton C with Birch K, Hunt K and Jordan K (1998) *Competition and Planning in the NHS* (2e). Stanley Thornes, Cheltenham.

Poole W (1999) *The need for longitudinal assessments of patient compliance*. Presentation to the HSMU, Manchester.

Poole W and Birch K (1996) *Local Delivery*. Centre for Health Planning and Management, University of Keele.

Poole W and Birch K (1997) *Mothers and Midwives*. Centre for Health Planning and Management, University of Keele.

Rigby M (ed) (2000) *Taking Health Telematics into the 21st Century*. Radcliffe Medical Press, Oxford.

Roberts JS, James S and Regina M (1984) Towards effective quality assurance: the evolution and current standards of the JCAH QA standard. *Quality Review Bulletin* 10(1): 11–15.

Roberts R (1999) *Information for Evidence-Based Care*. Radcliffe Medical Press, Oxford.

Rodger E and Watkins S (1999) Variations enigma. *Health Service Journal* 109: 20–3.

Roland M (1997) Presentation to Royal College of General Practitioners Conference 14 November 1997, *Measuring General Practice*.

Roland M, Holden J and Campbell S (1998) *Quality Assessment for General Practice: supporting clinical governance in primary care groups*. NPCRDC, Manchester.

Rosenthal MM (1995) *The Incompetent Doctor: behind closed doors*. Open University Press, Buckingham.

Rust RT and Oliver RL (1994) *Service Quality*. Sage, London.

Scally G and Donaldson L (1998) Clinical governance and the drive for quality improvement in the new NHS in England. *BMJ*. 317: 61–5.

ScHARR (1997) *Measures to Assist GPs Whose Performance Gives Cause for Concern*. University of Sheffield.

Scrivens E (1995) *Accreditation: protecting the professional or consumer?* Open University Press, Buckingham.

Scrivens E (1998) *A Scoping Study for Clinical Governance in Primary Care* (Report for the Department of Health). Centre for Health Planning and Management, University of Keele.

Scrivens E, Birch K and Gegios A (2000) *An Evaluation of Two Locally-Developed Accreditation Programmes.* Centre for Health Planning and Management, University of Keele.

Scrivens E and Blaylock P (1997) *Developments in Accreditation in Primary Care.* ISQua, Victoria, Australia.

Sheldon T (1998) Promoting health care quality: what role performance indicators. *Quality in Health Care* December supplement: 45–50.

Shields Report (1996) *Commissioning Better Health: Report of Short Life Working Group on the Roles and Responsibilities of Health Boards.* Scottish Office, Edinburgh.

Starfield B (1998) Quality of care research: internal elegance and external relevance. *JAMA.* **Sept 16:** 1006.

Teixeira J *et al.* (1999) Association between maternal anxiety in pregnancy and increased uterine artery resistance index: cohort based study. *BMJ.* **318:** 153–7.

The Patient's Network (1998) *Moving Patients to the Center of Health Care* 3(3).

Further reading

Allsop J and Mulchaey L (1996) *Regulating Medical Work: formal and informal controls.* Open University Press, Buckingham.

Audit Commission (1996) *What the Doctor Ordered: a study of GPFH in England and Wales.* The Stationery Office, London.

Donabedian A (1979) The quality of medical care: a concept in search of a definition. *Family Practitioner* **9:** 277–84.

Donabedian A (1981) Criteria, norms and standards of quality: what do they mean? *American Journal of Public Health* **71:** 409–12.

Moussa A and Webb C (1994) Quality of care in general practice: a Delphi study of indicators and methods. *Australian Family Physician* **23(3):** 465–8.

Øvretveit J (1992) *Health Service Quality.* Blackwell, Oxford.

Pollitt C (1993) The politics of medical quality: auditing doctors in the UK and USA. *Health Services Management Research* **6:** 1.

Rosenthal MM, Mulcahy L and Lloyd-Bostock S (eds) (1999) *Medical Mishaps: pieces of the puzzle.* Open University Press, Buckingham.

Scrivens E (1997) The impact of accreditation systems upon patient care. *Journal of Clinical Effectiveness* 2(4).

Toon PD (1994) *What is Good General Practice?* RCGP, London.

Webb PJC (1995) *Primary Care Accreditation.* Health Services Accreditation, London.

Index

Milton Keynes UK
Ingram Content Group UK Ltd.
UKHW031150141024
449569UK00024B/927

9 781857 753646